Top Tips in Critical Care

Edited by

G R Park
Director of Intensive Care Research
Addenbrooke's NHS Trust
Cambridge
UK

Rob Sladen
Professor of Anaesthesia
Columbia University
New York
USA

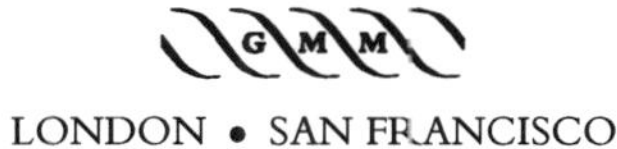

LONDON • SAN FRANCISCO

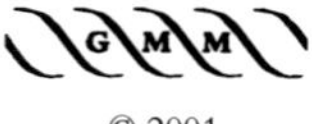

Greenwich Medical Media Limited
137 Euston Road
London NW1 2AA

870 Market Street, Ste 720,
San Francisco, CA 94102

ISBN 1 84110 120 6

First Published 2001

While the advice and information in this book is believed to be true and accurate, neither the authors nor the publisher can accept responsibility or liability for any loss or damage arising from actions or decisions based in this book. The ultimate responsibility for treatment of patients and the interpretation lies with the medical practitioner. The opinions expressed are those of the author and the inclusion in the book of information relating to a particular product, method of technique does not amount to an endorsement of its value or quality, or of the claims made of it by its manufacturers. Every effort has been made to check drug dosages: however, it is still possible that errors have occurred. Furthermore, dosage schedules are constantly being revised and new side effects recognised. For these reasons, the medical practitioners is strongly urged to consult the drug companies' printed instructions before administering any of the drugs mentioned in the book.

The publisher makes no representation, express or implied, with regard to the accuracy of the information contained in this book and cannot accept any legal responsibility or liability for any errors or omissions that may be made.

A catalogue record for this book is available from the British Library.

Project Manager
Gavin Smith

Typeset by Charon Tec Pvt. Ltd, Chennai, India

Printed in the UK by the Alden Group

Distributed by Plymbridge Distributors Ltd and
in the USA by Jamco Distribution

Visit our website at: **www.greenwich-medical.co.uk**

CONTENTS

PREFACE

Critical care is a complex and technical specialty. As time goes by, every practitioner starts to find useful and common sense ways to deal with difficult and challenging situations. Many of these "tips" (how to do it) and "caveats" (how not to do it!) are passed on by word of mouth to colleagues, juniors and others. Most of them are not "big" enough to warrant publication in journals and so remain part of our oral medical history, some surviving only within a single unit or institution. This small book aims to enable these tips to be shared amongst a much wider audience.

Some readers might opine that this book is the very antithesis of the current trend for evidence based medicine. They are right. But even in critical care medicine there remains a need for skill and artistry based upon cumulative — and often hard-won — experience. It is this legacy that this book explores.

Other readers may consider some of the tips obvious and basic. Indeed some are, but we all have to learn these at some stage. Hopefully this book will appeal to both novices and experts.

For the editors it has been a fascinating experience sifting through so many tips received from practitioners all over the world. We don't necessarily agree with them all, that is something for the reader to decide. What may be accepted practice in the UK or Europe may be anathema to a North American practitioner, and vice versa. Nor do we accept responsibility for the usefulness or safety of these tips — that remains with the contributor. We have, therefore, rejected very few and hope that the reader will intelligently evaluate each tip before using them on patients!

Personal experience is never static, but constantly grows and expands. By the same token, when you have read this book you may feel you have tips (and caveats) to offer, too. Please send them to one of the authors: when we have enough new ones we will publish a second edition!

G R PARK
Cambridge, UK
gilbertpark@compuserve.com

R N SLADEN
New York, USA
rs543@columbia.edu

CONTRIBUTORS

J Aman, South Africa
N Appleyard, Sheffield, UK
A R Bodenham, Leeds, UK
C Brown, Manchester, UK
D B Coursin, Madison, USA
C Clinton, Johannesburg, South Africa
A J Coe, Scunthorpe, UK
N Cohen, San Francisco, USA
D Coursin, Madison, USA
M Farrington, Cambridge, UK
J Gannon, Wirral, UK
K E Gunning, Cambridge, UK
M Heath, New York, USA
P Lawler, Middlesbrough, UK
M J Lindop, Cambridge, UK
P B Lumb, Albany, USA
D MacGregor, Winston-Salem, USA
B Matta, Cambridge, UK
J O'Hanlon, Belfast, Ireland
G R Park, Cambridge, UK
M L Pepperman, Leicester, UK
S Ridley, Norwich, UK
D W Ryan, Newcastle-upon-Tyne, UK
M P Shelly, Manchester, UK

M Singer, London, UK

G Skowronski, Australia

R Sladen, New York, USA

J L van der Spoel, Netherlands

T Welchew, Sheffield, UK

A White, Milton Keynes, UK

P V Woodsford, Glamorgan, Wales

D F Zandstra, Netherlands

CHAPTER 1

AIRWAY MANAGEMENT

Tracheostomy

"Minitrach"

Minitracheostomy provides two challenges: the risk of incorrect placement and bleeding.

Tip:

- Visualizing the trachea using the intubating laryngoscope can reduce the risk of misplacement.
- First, infiltrate down to the insertion site and into the trachea using bupivacaine with adrenaline (epinephrine) to reduce bleeding.
- On entering trachea with the needle, aspirate air into this same solution, then instill 2 mL of bupivacaine into the trachea to prevent coughing.
- If bleeding persists it can be controlled with tension sutures placed laterally.

D W Ryan, Newcastle-upon-Tyne, UK

Emergency cricothyroidotomy

If you perform an emergency cricothyroidotomy, you may have to ventilate the patient through a large needle (14 gauge or larger calibre), or an 8 French flexible catheter.

Tip:

As a make-shift adaptor, remove the barrel from a 3 mL syringe and attach the syringe to the needle or catheter. The adaptor from a 7.0 mm tracheal tube will fit and attach to a self-inflating bag allowing ventilation of the lungs.

D B Coursin, Madison, Wisconsin, USA

Fibreoptic assisted percutaneous tracheostomy

Because percutaneous tracheostomy is a relatively "blind" procedure, it is important to ensure correct placement of the seeker needle and dilators.

Tip:

A fibreoptic bronchoscope placed via the endotracheal tube can be used to confirm correct placement of the needle and dilator during percutaneous tracheostomy.

Caveat:

There is a significant reduction in ventilation when the bronchoscope is in the endotracheal tube, and while this may not be sufficient to affect oxygenation, it may increase $PaCO_2$. This is detrimental in situations where hypercarbia must be avoided, such as in patients with elevated intracranial pressure.

B Matta, Cambridge, UK

Tip:

In non-intubated patients undergoing percutaneous tracheostomy, consider using a laryngeal mask airway with the fibrescope inserted through it to maintain ventilation during the procedure.

M J Lindop, Cambridge, UK

Tracheostomy reinsertion

Changing the tracheostomy tube within the first 5 days after percutaneous tracheostomy may be hazardous because it is unlikely that a secure tract will have yet formed.

Tip:

- Use a non-cuffed paediatric endotracheal tube as a guide.
- Select a size that just fits through the tube that you wish to insert — NOT the one that you are about to take out — assuming that you are changing for a tube of similar size or smaller.
- Cut about 1.5 cm off the connector end of the paediatric tracheal tube (this is often slightly wider to take the connector).
- Use this paediatric endotracheal tube as a guide.
- If you can't find an uncuffed endotracheal tube then cutting the cuff (and pilot tube) off a cuffed version works almost as well — but take care you don't lose it down the trachea!

N Appleyard, Sheffield, UK

Tip:

Instead of using dilating forceps, a soft bronchial suction catheter introduced through the tracheostome will guide the tracheostomy tube into the right place.

S Ridley, Norwich, UK

Nasotracheal intubation

This is not always easy. Some of the problems include:

- epistaxis on insertion
- inability to pass through nasal passages
- nasotracheal tubes may cause pressure necrosis of the external nares.

Tip:

To overcome these difficulties, prepare the nose with 10% cocaine paste to diminish bleeding. Ensure that the nose is patent, and septum not deviated by using a gloved index finger.

If the tracheal tube cannot pass beyond the soft palate place a gloved finger into the post nasal space and place the end of the tube onto the finger, from where it can be manoeuvred into the pharynx.

Always use an uncut tube to prevent damage to the nares and allow the tube to dangle, thereby avoiding traction and torque on the nose.

D W Ryan, Newcastle-upon-Tyne, UK

With oral intubation, the size of the laryngeal aperture defines the maximum size of the tracheal tube.

Tip:

As a rough guide, the laryngeal aperture is the same diameter as the patient's little finger.

For nasotracheal intubation, the narrowest part of the airway is not the laryngeal aperture, but the nasal passage. Choosing the largest nasal passage is important.

▼

Tip:

As a generalisation, the nasal septum always deviates: choose the narrowest anterior nasal passage — the septum deviates away making the posterior aperture above the soft palate bigger. You can dilate the nasal passage by putting your gloved finger in the narrowest nasal passage and the twisting your finger in the nares: the proximal, or distalinter-phalyngeal joint acts as the dilator. Because the rotational movement may be painful for you, you will be reltively gentle.

P Lawler, Middlesbrough, UK

Blind nasal intubation

With the advent of the laryngeal mask airway, blind nasal intubation has become something of a "lost art". Nonetheless, it can be an expedient means of tracheal intubation in a patient in acute respiratory distress who is unable and/or unwilling to open their mouth. It facilitates airway management with the need for little or no central sedation in hemodynamically unstable patients, and obviates the need to control ventilation in a patient who is "air hungry" and has a high minute ventilation. Indeed, blind nasal intubation is easiest in patients with severe air hunger, whose respiratory efforts dilate the trachea and literally suck the tube in!

Caveats:

The presence of a coagulopathy or anticoagulation is an absolute contraindication to nasal intubation. Death may be caused in such a patient by massive epistaxis and asphyxiation.

Although nasotracheal intubation has its adherents, in particular because the tube is more stable and the patient cannot bite down on it, it has a number of limitations. Often a smaller tube has to be used than would be placed via the orotracheal route, which limits suctioning access. Its longer length and curve through the nasopharynx make it more liable to occlusion by mucus.

The most compelling argument against the routine use of nasotracheal intubation is that there is good evidence that the nasopharynx becomes contaminated by nosocomial (often Gram-negative) organisms within 48 hours, and thereafter serves as a constant reservoir for sinusitis and systemic infection. So even if nasotracheal intubation is the most expeditious route for emergency airway management, I recommend changing it to the oral route — if this can be safely accomplished — within 48 hours.

Tip:

In any event, here are a few tips for successful blind nasal intubation in an awake, unintubated patient:

1. Explain to the patient — if they are able to understand — exactly what you are about to do.
2. Soak several cotton-tips in 4% cocaine. Gently introduce one into the nares, and leave in position for a minute or two. Then add another, advancing it a little further into the nose. Repeat this procedure, removing the superficial cotton-tips, until the angle of the nasopharynx has been turned. Reassure the patient — cocaine burns! But it accomplishes two very important things:
   - local anaesthesia; and
   - intense mucosal vasoconstriction.

[If cocaine is contraindicated by the patient's cardiac status, dilute phenylephrine can be a safe, although a less effective vasoconstrictor.]

3. While you are waiting for the cocaine to take effect, hold the distal end of the endotracheal tube under a running hot water tap. This will soften it, and make it easier to pass through the nose. Lubricate it well with lidocaine (lignocaine) jelly.
4. Place the patient's head into the "sniffing position" [this adage applies to all attempts at tracheal intubation, blind or direct]. First, flex the neck by placing a pillow or towel under occiput. Then, extend the head on the neck. Correct positioning of the head can make or break an attempt at tracheal intubation.
5. Insert the tube into the larger nostril. Use gentle, firm and continuous pressure. If the nares is too tight, withdraw and try the other nostril. The tube should never be forced through the nose because turbinates can easily be torn off, and attempts should be abandoned if excessive resistance is encountered. Try a smaller tube.
6. As the tube nears the glottis, you will become aware of condensation in the tube with each exhalation. Position your head close to the patient, listen to the breath sounds and watch the patient's chest. As the tube gets closer still to the glottis, you will hear a harsh expiratory breath sound in the tube. Slowly position the tube until that sound is loudest. Loss of sound means that you have come up against the glottis, vallecula or gone into the esophagus.
7. Now comes the *coup de grace*. Your timing and deftness of thrust should equal that of a skilled matador. Watch the chest move and listen to the tracheal sound. Just as the patient starts a breath, give the tube a quick downward thrust.

8. Successful tracheal intubation is unmistakeable — there is no resistance to downward motion of the tube, and breath sounds (plus or minus tracheal secretions) emanate from it. Beware — oesophageal intubation causes little resistance either! Correct tracheal positioning can be confirmed by auscultation of the lungs and over the stomach while giving positive pressure breaths, or by using a capnograph.

If you meet a "rubbery" resistance to the tube with downward movement, do not persist — the tube has abutted against the epiglottis or vallecula. Withdraw until the breath sounds are harshest again, position the head slightly left or right, up or down (trying to achieve still louder breath sounds) then try again. Occasionally it is necessary to resort to direct laryngoscopy and assistance in positioning with a Magill forceps. Mind that you don't tear the cuff with this manoeuvre!

R N Sladen, New York, USA

Protecting the cuff on a nasotracheal tube

Pushing a cuffed nasotracheal tube through the nares can damage or puncture the cuff as it is pushed or snags against the inferior conchae (which are often sharp).

Tip:

When you have pushed the tube through into the nasopharynx, always check the cuff. The cuff can be protected by cutting off a glove finger and pushing it over the tip of the tube to cover the cuff (acting as a finger stall). The "finger" must be rescued using Magill forceps when it has passed through into the oropharynx. Forgetting to remove this finger stall is dangerous!

P Lawler, Middlesbrough, UK

Nasotracheal tube security

Once inserted, nasotracheal tubes are tolerated much more readily by patients than orotracheal tubes. However, they are difficult to secure and need two tapes passing above and below the ears to stop them rolling forwards and downwards. These tapes have to be reasonably tight and are not tolerated very well by patients, as they tend to cut into the upper or lower part of the ear or pull the tube to one side or another.

Tip:

Pass a paediatric nasogastric tube gently through one nostril, around the posterior nasal septum and back through the other nostril to secure the nasotracheal tube. This manoeuvre does away with the tapes, keeps the tube central and makes it impossible to pull the nasotracheal tube out without the patient becoming very uncomfortable. We have used this method for a wide variety of patients; from neonates to adult.

Tip:

Before passing a nasotracheal tube, the nasogastric tube is passed through one nostril into the oropharynx and brought out of the mouth using a laryngoscope and Magill forceps. A suitable suction catheter is passed via the other nostril and brought out in the mouth. The nasogastric tube is attached to the suction catheter by pushing one inside the other and the suction catheter pulled back out of its nostril bringing the tip of the nasogastric tube with it. The two ends of the nasogastric tube are then tied together with a reef knot.

The patient is then re-intubated with a nasotracheal tube and the nasogastric tube used to tie the nasotracheal tube in place.

P V Woodsford, Glamorgan, Wales

Directing the nasotracheal tube

When the tube is being pushed through the nose, it follows the floor of the nasal cavity. As it emerges from the posterior nasal space, the tube may fail to turn down into the oropharynx because it gets caught on the second intervertebral cartilage, particularly in elderly, osteoarthritic patients.

Tip:

Several manoeuvres may help:

- First, push the head back (i.e. extending the head on the atlanto-occipital joint): this may improve the entry
- Next, rotate the tube in a corkscrew motion
- Finally, you may have to put your finger in the mouth and hook the tube forward

If all else fails, and you must insert a nasotracheal tube e.g. in someone who may have an epileptic fit (seizure) or is biting the tube, put in a nasogastric tube, fish this out of the mouth, and use this as a guide to railroad the tube into the mouth, and "round the corner".

P Lawler, Middlesbrough, UK

Lost nasotracheal tube

On occasions you can push the endotracheal tube onwards beyond the nasopharynx, but it can't be identified by direct laryngoscopy. The tube will have pierced the mucosa in the posterior nasopharyngeal wall and is burrowing underneath it, in the potential space between nasopharynx and fascia covering the vertebral column. Sometimes the tube emerges in the posterior oropharynx.

Tip:

If you suspect this is the case, remove the tube and start again, using your fingers to guide the tube into the oropharynx (as above). If you have covered the tip of the tube with a finger stall, make sure you do not lose it in this space.

P Lawler, Middlesbrough, UK

Difficulty intubating the trachea

The nasotracheal tube may be difficult to place in the larynx. This occurs because the shape of the nasopharynx directs the tube in an anterior direction. The result is that the tube may catch on the anterior commissure at the anterior junction of the vocal cords, just beneath the epiglottis.

Tip:

With the tube pushed into the anterior commissure, the head is flexed on the atlanto-occipital joint. This carries the tube posteriorly, so it may slip into the laryngeal aperture.

Either combined with this manoeuvre, or separately, the tube should be rotated, so that it "corkscrews" into the larynx: the standard position of the bevel helps this corkscrew manoeuvre.

P Lawler, Middlesbrough, UK

Tracheal tubes with Murphy eyes

The "eye" can be a problem during percutaneous tracheostomy because the introducing needle and wire may inadvertently be placed through it.

Tip:

Always check the position of the guidewire and first introducer with a fibreoptic bronchoscope.

P Lawler, Middlesbrough, UK

Tracheal intubation in patients with rheumatoid arthritis

Patients with rheumatoid arthritis involving the cervical spine and temporomandibular joints present a major challenge in securing the airway:

- Usually have a full set of prominent teeth.
- They cannot fully open their mouths.
- A small mandible pushes the normal-sized tongue backwards into the upper pharynx, making the airway very narrow antero-posteriorly.
- Osteophytes and inflammation of the bodies of the cervical vertebrae push anteriorly, making the airway even more narrow antero-posteriorly, and displacing the tracheal inlet anteriorly as well.
- There is usually a degree of fixed flexion of the neck, which may be severe.
- If the cervical vertebrae show any signs or symptoms of subluxation, then the neck will need to be fixed in a comfortable position before general anaesthesia can be contemplated.

Caveats:

Flexible, fiberoptic intubation is probably the technique of choice. Unfortunately, this is made more difficult by the very anterior larynx and fixed flexion deformity, which together may make the laryngeal inlet exquisitely difficult to reach with the fiberoptic laryngoscope. This problem is compounded by the antero-posteriorly narrow pharynx, which hinders visualising the anatomy in the awake patient, and which tends to collapse and obstruct the airway when the patient is anaesthetised.

Traditionally, a gaseous (inhalation) induction has been used for these patients. However, the anaesthetic may cause its own airway problems such as coughing or laryngospasm. Also, as soon as an airway problem occurs, the level of anaesthesia lightens, whilst the patient becomes hypoxic. The combination of stage 2 anaesthesia, a very difficult airway and hypoxia cannot be considered elements of a "safe" technique.

Tip:

Let the patient breath 100% oxygen and start a propofol infusion at approximately 100 mL/hr (about 200 μgs/kg/min in an 80 kg patient) and adjusted according to response. Patients drift off to sleep over 3–4 minutes. If there is an airway problem, the propofol can be turned off in the same way that a gas (inhalation) induction is stopped. There is unlikely to be laryngospasm using this technique because only oxygen gets to the airway.

The next "trick" solves the problem of the collapsing airway and the anterior larynx in these patients.

Tip:

Load an uncut plain 5.5 mm endotracheal tube onto the fibreoptic laryngoscope. When the patient is anaesthetised, pass a size 2.5 laryngeal mask (small size because these patients have small upper airways) into the patient's airway. This can be used to keep the airway open, despite its tendency to collapse. Pass the fibreoptic laryngoscope down the laryngeal mask and through the central fenestration. The laryngeal mask splints the narrow upper airway open, whilst its built-in curvature carries the laryngoscope anteriorly in a way it cannot do on its own. The epiglottis and larynx can be found in the usual way. If not, the laryngeal mask probably needs to be reinserted again. Having entered the trachea with the laryngoscope, the 5.5 mm tracheal tube can be railroaded down and will pass through the central fenestration of the laryngeal mask into the trachea without alteration to either tube or laryngeal mask.

T Welchew, Sheffield, UK

Airway management in patients with severe cervical spine problems

Tip:

Unless the patient needs ventilating, allow the patient to breathe spontaneously whilst insufflating gaseous anaesthetic agents from the oropharynx. These can be delivered through a nasopharyngeal airway. The patient's lips may have to be taped together to maintain the reservoir of anaesthetic agents in the oropharynx.

M L Pepperman, Leicester, UK

Identifying the position of the endotracheal tube

A frequent occurrence in the ICU is the approach of a resident bearing a chest X-ray and asking "what do you think about the position of the endotracheal tube?". Long before the chest X-ray is taken, the resident should be taken to the bedside and taught about "bouncing the cuff".

Tip:

The key element of the procedure is that the practitioner applies intermittent pressure to the pilot balloon, while feeling the trachea above the suprasternal notch. When the pilot balloon is squeezed, the pressure (and position) of the expanding cuff will be felt by the observer's fingers.

This procedure tells you if the endotracheal tube is too high or too low, but does not discern between tracheal vs esophageal placement — however, I have to assume that you would have found that out already!

M Heath, New York, USA

Tracheal tube tolerance (1)

Some intubated patients wake up and cough on the tracheal tube, but may not be ready for extubation and you may be reluctant to re-sedate them (for example, their $PaCO_2$ is 55 mmHg [7.3 kPa]).

Tip:

Consider a trial of intravenous lidocaine (lignocaine). Administer 1 mg/kg slowly over about two to three minutes. There is a good chance that the patient will experience immediate and dramatic relief from irritation caused by the tracheal tube (some may even sleep for a while).

If the patient has a good response to the bolus, start an intravenous infusion of lidocaine at 2 mg/min. This can buy you the 1–3 hours the patient may need to be able to extubate the patient safely.

R N Sladen, New York, USA

Tip:

To reduce the amount of sedation some long-term patients need to tolerate the endotracheal tube, nebulised bupivicaine can be useful. We give 3 mL 0.5% bupivicaine without adrenaline up to hourly. If some of the coughing is caused by bleeding, the use of an adrenaline containing solution may help with this.

G R Park, Cambridge, UK

Changing an endotracheal tube

One of the problems encountered using an endotracheal tube changer is that the tube may become "hung up" at the epiglottis.

Tip:

When using an endotracheal tube changer, align the tip of the endotracheal tube so that it will slide under the epiglottis. If you meet resistance, rotate the endotracheal tube 90° and try again. If this does not work, try again. If that fails, try using a smaller endotracheal tube.

Tip:

Alternatively, for a difficult endotracheal tube change, consider using the fiberoptic bronchoscope to place a second tube. Then place the fiberoptic bronchoscope into the original tube and pull it out under direct visualization. Use lots of lubrication or silicone spray on the outside of the new tube so it does not stick to the original one.

D B Coursin, Madison, Wisconsin, USA

CHAPTER 2

VENTILATION AND BLOOD GASES

BIPAP

BIPAP (bimodal positive airway pressure) is useful for decreasing work of breathing and preventing atelectasis in spontaneously breathing patients.

Caveat:

BIPAP should not be used in patients with abnormal intracranial compliance. The minute volume is very variable and any decrease may cause hypercarbia. This in turn increases intracranial blood flow and pressure, and diminishes cerebral perfusion pressure.

B Matta, Cambridge, UK

Adding up the arterial blood gases

The inspired oxygen concentration in % is almost the same as the partial pressure of oxygen in kPa: e.g. 35% oxygen is 35 kPa (at sea level!). This is an application of the alveolar air equation, the simplest rough and ready version of which says $P_IO_2 = PaO_2 + PaCO_2$.

Tip:

For arterial blood gases, always add up the $PaCO_2$ and the PaO_2. If the sum is much more than the inspired oxygen tension, then either the patient is getting more oxygen than you thought, or the blood gas machine is broken.

P Lawler, Middlesbrough, UK

Some PEEP caveats

Positive end-expiratory pressure (PEEP) remains the most frequent intervention used to provide airway pressure therapy for atelectasis, consolidation or pulmonary edema.

Caveat:

During pressure control ventilation, if tidal volume increases when extrinsic PEEP is decreased, it suggests that the lungs are being over-inflated.

The implication is that PEEP is causing air-trapping (excess Lung Zone 1). The increase in dead space comes at the expense of alveolar ventilation, which improves when PEEP is decreased. This scenario is most likely to occur in patients with emphysema or localized lung disease.

Caveat:

An increase in stroke volume with an increase in PEEP suggests intravascular volume overload. Conversely, a decrease in stroke volume suggests left ventricular underfilling.

In the former case, PEEP has decreased venous return to the heart, and relieved ventricular overdistension. In the latter, the decreased venous return to the heart has further decreased effective preload in a hypovolemic patient.

M Singer, London, UK

How much PEEP?

The optimum level or "best" PEEP is arguably that which converts noncompliant atelectatic lung units (Zone 3) to compliant lung units (Zone 2). However, excessive PEEP overdistends alveoli and again renders them noncompliant.

Tip:

The "best" PEEP could be defined as that which increases compliance most. During IPPV with a prolonged I-E ratio and measurable plateau pressure, an improvement in compliance when PEEP is added is reflected by its "absorption" into the plateau pressure. That is, if PEEP improves compliance, the plateau pressure would increase by less than the added PEEP.

In the following example, PEEP is added in increments of 3 cm H_2O:

PEEP 3	plateau pressure 33	net pressure (33 – 3) = 30
PEEP 6	plateau pressure 35	net pressure (35 – 6) = 29
PEEP 9	plateau pressure 36	net pressure (36 – 9) = 27
PEEP 12	plateau pressure 42	net pressure (42 – 12) = 30

"Best" PEEP is that with the smallest net increase in plateau pressure, i.e. 9.

P Lawler, Middlesbrough, UK

Ventilator adjustments and arterial blood gases

Patients on supplemental oxygen or mechanical ventilatory assistance should be assessed with respect to blood gas values predicted from the level of support provided.

Tip:

- To estimate the PaO_2 in mmHg, for an F_IO_2 of 0.21 increasing to 0.5, multiply F_IO_2 by 5
- To estimate the PaO_2 in mmHg, for an F_IO_2 of 0.5 increasing to 1.0, multiply F_IO_2 by 6

Therefore, a patient with normal lungs at an F_IO_2 of 0.4 is expected to have a PaO_2 of 200 mmHg.

The degree of ventilation — perfusion mismatch may be estimated by realizing that for each 15 mmHg discrepancy between the predicted and measured PaO_2 there is approximately a 1% intrapulmonary shunt.

P B Lumb, Albany, USA

Prediction of arterial blood gases based on ventilatory data

Tip:

To estimate the PaO_2, remember the normal values for the following variables:

- The normal dead space to tidal volume (V_d/V_t) ratio is 0.3
- Anatomic dead space in mL = patient weight in pounds
- Tracheal intubation decreases anatomic dead space between 30% and 50%
- Ventilator tube compliance is such that the tubing distends approximately 3–5 mL/cmH_2O inflation pressure
- The relationship between $PaCO_2$ and minute ventilation is linear within normal physiologic ranges.

With this information, the following example outlines appropriate management.

A 70 kg male 25 year old trauma victim is admitted to the Emergency Department. Mechanical ventilation is started with a 9.0 orotracheal tube and the patient is placed on positive pressure ventilation with the following settings:

F_IO_2	0.4
Tidal volume (V_t)	850 mL
Rate (frequency, f)	10 breaths/min
Peak inflation pressure (PIP)	20 cmH_2O

Predict the arterial blood gases assuming no significant chest trauma.

From the previous tip, the predicted PaO_2 is 200 mmHg.

$PaCO_2$ is slightly more difficult to estimate, but the following points may be helpful:

- A 70 kg adult has a alveolar minute ventilation of 4.0–5.0 L/min
- 70 kg = approximately 150 lbs, so the patient has 150 mL dead space
- If the V_d/V_t is normal (0.3), the tidal volume = 450 mL
- Alveolar ventilation/breath = 0.7 × 450 = 325 mL
- Average ventilatory rate = 14 breaths/min

Therefore, alveolar minute ventilation = 325 × 14 = 4.5 L/min.

Normally, this creates a $PaCO_2$ of 40 mmHg.

In the example above, the patient has a alveolar minute ventilation of 7.15 L/min.

The predicted $PaCO_2$ is 25 mmHg.

This is calculated as follows:

The set tidal volume was 850 mL.

The alveolar tidal volume is calculated by subtracting

(a) 75 mL dead space (half theoretical dead space because of the endotracheal tube), and
(b) 60 mL (the volume lost in the distended tubing, i.e. 3 mL × 20 cmH_2O PIP)

Thus, the alveolar tidal volume is 715 mL.

A ventilator rate of 10 breaths/min provides an alveolar minute ventilation of 7.15 L.

Therefore, the calculated

$$
\begin{aligned}
PaCO_2 &= 40 - (40 \times \{[7.15 - 4.5]/7.15\}) \\
&= 40 - (40 \times 0.37) \\
&= 40 - 15 \\
&= 25\,\text{mmHg}
\end{aligned}
$$

The calculations are important at the bedside in order to quantify the patient's support requirements and to avoid mistakes. No interpretation of blood gases should be performed without considering how it matches or differs from the predicted values.

P B Lumb, Albany, USA

Application of continuous positive airway pressure (CPAP)

In the spontaneously breathing patient, the application of CPAP provides positive end-expiratory pressure (PEEP) which can reverse or prevent atelectasis, improve functional residual capacity (FRC) and oxygenation, and possibly forestall the need tracheal intubation.

Caveat:

Mask CPAP (i.e. the application of CPAP via a tightly fitting face mask) requires endless adjustment of bandanna strapping and often is poorly tolerated by the patient.

Tip:

Nasal CPAP is easier to use and better tolerated. A specially designed small nasal mask applies CPAP but allows the patient to talk and cough.

Alternatively, a standard nasal airway can be inserted with same size tracheal tube catheter connection insert *in situ*. Then, using conventional circuitry, CPAP can then be attached to the patient.

D W Ryan, Newcastle-upon-Tyne, UK

Is CPAP flow sufficient?

If the CPAP circuit flow is insufficient to match the patient's peak inspiratory flow rate, the patient will breathe against a closed circuit. This creates negative intrapleural pressure and risks the development of pulmonary oedena.

Tip:

Always look at the expiratory valve in all patients on CPAP. The valve should always remain slightly open during inspiration. This ensures that the flow rate through the system is sufficient to match the patient's peak inspiratory flow rate.

G R Park, Cambridge, UK

Excess vagal tone

The occurrence of bradycardia during tracheal suction, endotracheal tube manipulation, or hand ventilation suggests the presence of dysautonomia.

Tip:

- Have some atropine handy.
- Make sure the patient does not have critically ill polyneuropathy: nerve conduction studies may be useful.
- Think whether weaning is appropriate at this time.

P Lawler, Middlesbrough, UK

Sudden change in gas exchange

Tip:

Always exclude a tension pneumothorax when the gas exchange in a patient receiving mechanical ventilation deteriorates suddenly.

K E Gunning, Cambridge, UK

Diagnosis of adult respiratory distress syndrome (ARDS)

The diagnosis of ARDS is based upon the development of acute respiratory failure associated with radiological pulmonary infiltrates and a pulmonary artery occlusion pressure (PAOP) less than 18 mmHg. However, heart failure or fluid overload may coexist with ARDS. If the PAOP is high how can one make a diagnosis of ARDS?

Tip:

- Measure the colloid oncotic pressure (COP, normally 20–25 mmHg) of pulmonary oedema fluid:
  - if it is low it is a transudate, i.e. suggestive of heart failure
  - if its high it is an exudate, i.e. suggestive of ARDS, infection etc.
- Perform a pulmonary occlusion angiogram, by injecting radiocontrast dye through a pulmonary artery catheter in the PAOP position: if its abnormal, the patient has ARDS

P Lawler, Middlesbrough, UK

Mechanical ventilation in acute asthma

There is a real danger in mechanical ventilation of asthmatic patients: excessive lung inflation or ventilator rate results in air trapping because the next breath is delivered before complete exhalation. This can result in "stacking" of breaths, hyperinflation, worsened hypercarbia and even tension pneumothorax.

Tip:

- Use a gentle hand ventilation after tracheal intubation, before mechanical ventilation is begun.
- Manual compression of the chest may be helpful in children to prevent air trapping.
- Measurement of the thoracic circumference, or disconnecting the patient from the ventilator intermittently, may reveal air trapping.
- Frequent (every 10 minutes) small aliquots of 0.9% saline instilled down the tracheal tube may loosen mucus plugs.

K E Gunning, Cambridge, UK

The inherent haemodynamic safety of hand ventilation for physiotherapy depends on the low airway pressures achievable with the bag. However, this will lead to under ventilation if the lungs are stiff or the airway resistance high. A simple "Water's" rubber bag cannot produce an airway pressure much greater than 30 cmH_2O. Airway pressures of this level are insufficient to ventilate patients with acute asthma (or even severe ARDS).

Tip:

Ventilation must be achieved either using a self inflating bag e.g. an Ambu bag, or the ventilator.

P Lawler, Middlesbrough, UK

Choice of drugs in asthmatic patients

Drugs which release histamine or block the β receptor can worsen bronchospasm in susceptible patients.

Caveat:

Avoid suxamethonium, atracurium, morphine, thiopentone, beta blockers, neostigmine.

Tip:

Use cisatracurium, rocuronium, vecuronium, fentanyl, propofol, ketamine.

G R Park, Cambridge, UK

Criteria for tracheal extubation

Prediction of successful tracheal extubation is usually straightforward, but in difficult patients, there is no one parameter that is always reliable. Single breath tests such as the forced vital capacity (FVC) >10 mL/kg and maximum inspiratory force (NIF) >−25 cmH_2O are useful measures of the patient's ability to cough and deep breathe, but do not predict work of breathing and endurance.

Tip:

The rapid shallow breathing index (frequency to tidal volume ratio, f/V_t) is easily performed on an awake, unsedated spontaneously breathing patient. It illustrates the ventilatory pattern, i.e. slow and deep, suggesting low work of breathing and success, or rapid and shallow, suggesting high work of breathing and failure.

The index is obtained by dividing the respiratory frequency in breaths/min by the tidal volume in litres. For example:

Frequency 20 breaths/min V_t 0.5 L
Index: 40 — predicts success

Frequency 24 breaths/min V_t 0.2 L
Index: 120 — predicts failure

P Lawler, Middlesbrough, UK

Hazards of tracheal intubation and positive pressure ventilation

Tracheal intubation, sedation and positive pressure ventilation of patients who are in acute respiratory failure and at the point of respiratory exhaustion will often cause marked hypotension, and occasionally even arrhythmias or cardiac arrest.

It is caused by dehydration secondary to inadequate fluid intake or forced diuresis (in an effort to improve pulmonary function), hyperventilation, and pyrexia.

Positive pressure ventilation decreases venous return to the heart and precipitously drops cardiac output. Sedation suppresses the high circulating catecholamine levels these stressed patients generate and induces relative peripheral vasodilation. The addition of muscle relaxants promotes pooling of blood in skeletal muscle (loss of the "muscle pump") and further decreases venous return to the heart.

Tip:

- Ensure that the patient has adequate intravenous access before intubation.
- Be ready to rapidly infuse fluids after intubation.
- Have a vasopressor (e.g. phenylephrine) ready to treat acute hypotension.
- Be cautious in the administration of sedative and relaxant drugs — give them in small, divided doses.
- Initiate ventilation with gentle hand ventilation. Convert to mechanical ventilation when the patient is more stable.

K E Gunning, Cambridge, UK
R N Sladen, New York, USA

Hazards in patients with end-stage obstructive lung disease

Tracheal intubation and mechanical ventilation in patients with end-stage chronic obstructive airways disease (COAD) [chronic obstructive pulmonary disease, COPD] presents all the hazards enumerated above and in addition, that of acute respiratory alkalosis, hypokalemia and arrhythmias. This is illustrated by the following example:

A 63-year old man with end-stage COPD has a baseline $PaCO_2$ of 58 mmHg [7.7 kPa]. With his compensatory metabolic alkolosis (bicarbonate 34 mEq/L) his pH is 7.36.

He develops acute bronchitis and respiratory failure, with an increase in $PaCO_2$ to 76 mmHg [10 kPa] and decrease in pH to 7.20. Serum potassium is 4.0 mEq/L.

You are called to intubate the patient because of acute distress and agonal breathing.

You do so without problem, place the patient on mechanical ventilation, and very soon thereafter the patient goes in to ventricular tachycardia. What has caused this shocking turn of events?

Tip:

An acute change in $PaCO_2$ of 10 mmHg [1.3 kPa] causes an acute change in pH of 0.08.

An acute change in pH of 0.1 causes an acute change in serum potassium of 0.5 mEq/L.

Based upon the above, ventilation to a $PaCO_2$ of 40 mmHg [5.3 kPa] would increase the pH by $(4 \times 0.08) = 0.32$, i.e. from 7.20 to 7.52.

A pH of 7.52 does not appear excessive, so why the sudden development of ventricular tachycardia?

The rapid increase in pH is associated with a marked intracellular flux of potassium. Thus, in the case above, the serum potassium will decrease by $(3.2 \times 0.5) = 1.6$ mEq/L, i.e. it will drop to 2.4 mEq/L.

The implication of a serum potassium of 4.0 mEq/L at a pH of 7.20 is total body hypokalemia. If the pH were corrected to 7.40, the serum potassium would be $4.0 - (2 \times 0.5 = 1.0)$, i.e. 3.0 mEq/L, most likely as a result of prior diuresis to "keep the lungs dry".

Tip:

Immediately after intubating a patient like the one described above, use gentle, assisted manual ventilation. Then, set up a level of mechanical ventilatory support designed to slowly correct the $PaCO_2$ toward baseline, i.e. 58 mmHg [7.7 kPa]. The patient will require also fluid administration and potassium supplementation.

R N Sladen, New York, USA

Suxamethonium (succinyl choline)

Patients on prolonged positive pressure ventilatory support commonly have developed a polyneuropathy or extra-junctional acetylcholine receptors.

Caveat:

Do not use suxamethonium (succinyl choline) as a muscle relaxant in patients who have had a prolonged ICU stay. It could cause massive discharge of potassium from muscle, and cardiac arrest.

P Lawler, Middlesbrough, UK

Bag or "bagging" the patient

Tip:

Try to avoid using this term. Conscious patients, when they hear it being used about them, may misconstrue it, causing distress.

G R Park, Cambridge, UK

Wheezing

In surgical patients, a common cause of wheezing is fluid overload ("cardiac asthma").

Tip:

It responds to diuretics!

G R Park, Cambridge, UK

Complications of chest drain insertion

During chest drain (pleural tube) insertion, impaling the lung with the tube in the lung is commoner than a bronchopleural fistula. Regrettably this can happen no matter how careful you are.

Tip:

If vigorous bubbling (air leak) persists for many hours after a chest drain is inserted, do a CT scan of the chest.

M J Lindop, Cambridge, UK

CHAPTER 3

CARDIOVASCULAR SYSTEM

Resuscitation

Pulmonary embolus

In pulmonary embolism blood pressure decreases because of impeded venous return to the left atrium.

Tip:

Lie the patient flat. The increase in venous return improves their cardiac output far more than sitting the patient up to aid their breathing.

M Singer, London, UK

Mask ventilation during cardiopulmonary resuscitation

In a patient with dentures, removal leads to loss of facial contours and may make a seal with a face mask difficult to achieve

Tip:

Find the patient's dentures and put them back in. If the dentures are reasonably well-fitting, the facial contours are restored and the mask fits a lot better. A Guedel airway also fits better.

P Lawler, Middlesbrough, UK

Caveat:

Remember to take the dentures out again before tracheal intubation!

R N Sladen, New York, USA

Cardiac arrhythmias

Tip:

Tachyarrhythmias and/or tachycardias which start on initiation of an inotropic or pressor agent usually imply ventricular underfilling. An empty heart is an irritable heart!

M Singer, London, UK

Heart failure

Heart failure may exist despite a high cardiac output.

Tip:

Give a fluid challenge — a gelatin or starch infusion — and re-measure the cardiac output and pulmonary artery occlusion pressure. Look at the change in left ventricular stroke work index and compare the increment with the normal. An impaired "slope" indicates a failing heart.

P Lawler, Middlesbrough, UK

Differential diagnosis of hypotension

Tip:

If a patient is hypotensive without an obvious cause, always exclude cardiac tamponade, occult bleeding or a tension pneumothorax.

K E Gunning, Cambridge, UK

Revealing hypovolaemia in vasoconstricted patients

Evaluation of intravascular hypovolaemia — even with invasive haemodynamic monitoring — may be obscured by the existence of intense arterial or venoconstriction, which may elevate blood pressure and cardiac filling pressures.

Tip:

A "nitrate challenge" is a useful and short-acting test for excessive arterial and/or venoconstriction. Dilute 5 mg glyceryl trinitrate in 20 mL saline (250 μg/mL). Give a bolus of 0.25–0.5 mL (62.5–125 μg).

- A decrease in blood pressure >15 mmHg suggests hypovolaemia.
- A decrease in blood pressure <15 mmHg and a decrease in stroke volume suggests arterial constriction and some underfilling.
- No change (or a small decrease) in blood pressure and an increase in stroke volume suggests arterial constriction, but reasonable filling.

M Singer, London, UK

Hypovolaemia and the arterial waveform

Early detection of hypovolaemia is important in many situations.

Tip:

The arterial trace may reveal the intravascular fluid depletion by an exaggeration of the decrease in pressure (pulsus paradoxus) that normally occurs during or shortly after inspiration. It may occur even before parameters such as central venous pressure, blood pressure or urine output substantially decrease, in both ventilated or spontaneously breathing patients.

A White, Milton Keynes, UK

Observation of haemodynamic trends

A single measurement of central venous pressure or pulmonary artery occlusion pressure (PAOP) may not define whether a given filling pressure is optimal for the patient's heart. For example, a PAOP of 5 mmHg may be adequate for a normal heart but totally inadequate for a poorly contractile heart.

Tip:

Use sequential fluid challenges to define a Starling curve for the heart and learn more about its contractile state and optimal filling pressure.

For example, following a fluid challenge of 1.5 mL/kg, an increase in the CVP of 2 cmH_2O or less indicates that the patient is intravascularly depleted, whilst an increase of 5 cm H_2O or more indicates the patient is fluid overloaded. Changes between 2 and 5 cm H_2O are equivocal.

Thus, resuscitation can be effected with relatively small volumes if the process is repeated until the increase in CVP is greater than 2 cmH_2O after any individual challenge.

If a pulmonary artery catheter is in place, the response of cardiac output to a fluid challenge provides even more meaningful information about the heart's contractile state and the ideal filling pressure. In a patient with low cardiac output and low filling pressures, sequential fluid challenges should be given until the cardiac output no longer increases (i.e. the flat portion of the Starling curve has been reached) or there is evidence of pulmonary congestion.

A White, Milton Keynes, UK
R N Sladen, New York, USA

Positioning to treat hypotension

The Trendelenberg (i.e. head down) position is frequently used to treat acute hypotension caused by hypovolemia in the early postoperative period. Venous return to the heart is rapidly augmented and hypovolemic hypotension rapidly improves while fluid are being infused or pressors administered. However, a steep Trendelenberg position markedly increases cerebral venous and intracranial pressure. This may be dangerous in some patients, for example those with a head injury.

Tip:

The same haemodynamic benefit can be achieved without compromise of cerebral perfusion pressure by simply elevating the supine patient's legs.

R N Sladen, New York, USA

Positioning to treat hypertension

Severe acute hypertension (e.g. rebound after sudden stopping of a sodium nitroprusside infusion) can precipitate cerebral hemorrhage or cardiac ischemia.

Tip:

Elevation of the head of the bed, or Reverse Trendelenberg position, can decrease blood pressure by venous pooling in the legs, as well as decrease the effective pressure in the brain and heart. The bed can be flattened once the appropriate pharmacologic intervention takes effect.

R N Sladen, New York, USA

Staff shift changes

Beware changes in any haemodynamic measurements at 07.00, 14.00, 21.00 h or whenever there is a change in nurse or doctor shifts — they may not be real changes, but result from a change in the transducer or bed position.

Tip:

Re-zero all transducers after staff shift changes!

P Lawler, Middlesbrough, UK

Response to labetalol

Labetalol is a unique and effective antihypertensive agent which combines α- and β-blockade. Initial dosing in the ICU requires careful titration, starting with as little as 2.5 mg iv, and then doubling the dose every 5–10 minutes until the desired effect is achieved.

Because of its β-blocking action, labetalol is most appropriate in patients with a heart rate of greater than 90 beats/min. The antihypertensive effect of labetolol takes about five minutes to work.

Tip:

Within about two minutes of labetalol injection a slowing of the heart rate is seen that is predictive of lowering of blood pressure response. If the heart rate does not change, it is unlikely that there will be a blood pressure response. This knowledge can save a considerable amount of time in titrating the effective dose of labetalol.

R N Sladen, New York, USA

CHAPTER 4

MONITORING

Pulmonary artery catheters

Inserting a pulmonary artery catheter (1)

When inserting a pulmonary artery catheter, it is important to maintain a three-dimensional awareness of the catheter tip in relationship to the anatomical structures through which it passes.

Tip:

Catheter length markings should be observed during the procedure. The right ventricle is usually entered between 25 and 35 cm from the right internal jugular vein. When the catheter enters the right ventricle, try to appreciate the gentle tug of the tricuspid valve as the balloon passes through it.

In order to avoid the potential complication of a kinked catheter, the pulmonary artery catheter should not be advanced more than 20 cm into the right ventricle without passing into the pulmonary artery. This is a useful safety check, although occasionally a patient with a dilated right ventricle requires greater insertion length. This should be appreciated before catheter manipulation.

During the procedure, ensure that there is adequate sterile pulmonary artery catheter with which to uncoil the catheter. Remember, if the coil is held in the hands during insertion, it is much easier to lose appreciation of tip orientation and direction.

P B Lumb, Albany, New York, USA

Inserting a pulmonary artery catheter (2)

Always make sure that the curve of the pulmonary artery catheter is going in the direction you want it to go (i.e. up the pulmonary artery).

Tip:

From the right internal jugular vein (the straightest shot), the tip of the catheter should be curving to the patient's left. I use the same curve when passing it through the left internal jugular vein, because the introducer will make the initial right turn into the innominate vein, and from the left subclavian vein. Passage via the right subclavian vein represents more of a challenge. Initially, it may be necessary to have the curve going to the right (to negotiate the bend from the subclavian to the innominate vein) and then rotate the catheter clockwise to reverse the curve once it has entered the right atrium.

R N Sladen, New York, USA

Inserting a pulmonary artery catheter (3)

Catheters are more difficult to pass with low cardiac output states.

Tip:

Consider increasing the dose of inotropic agents while inserting the catheter.

M J Lindop, Cambridge, UK

Inserting a pulmonary artery catheter (4)

During manufacture and storage, the pulmonary artery catheter develops a curl.

Tip:

Roll the catheter round your finger to offset the curl.

When attempting to float the catheter tip through the heart, always roll the catheter between your fingers (like a pencil) to encourage forward movement and stop snagging.

S Ridley, Norwich, UK

Difficult pulmonary artery catheter insertion (1)

Difficulty with placement of a pulmonary artery catheter may be encountered in the patient on mechanical ventilation, particularly during pressure control ventilation.

Tip:

Try advancing the catheter only during the expiratory phase of ventilation. This takes advantage of the increase in venous return to the heart that occurs during this phase of the ventilatory cycle, and is often successful when other attempts have failed.

C Clinton, Johannesburg, Gauteng, South Africa

Difficult pulmonary artery catheter insertion (2)

If you have been struggling to float a pulmonary artery catheter for more than five minutes and you are getting nowhere, stop. In the body, the catheter rapidly gets warmed to body temperature. This makes it very floppy and more likely to curl up in the right ventricle and elsewhere.

Tip:

Take the catheter out and flush it with cold saline. Wait two or three minutes. This lets the catheter and you cool down. Cooling down the catheter to room temperature makes it stiffer and less likely to curl up. Letting you cool down means that you can look at the patient and re-assess their status before you start again.

G R Park, Cambridge, UK

Difficult pulmonary artery catheter insertion (3)

While placement of a flow-directed pulmonary artery catheter usually proceeds smoothly, in some patients the catheter appears prone to curl up in the right ventricle. This occurs not infrequently in patients with enlarged ventricles, atrial fibrillation, regurgitant valves, or low flow states.

Tip:

In this situation I find it very helpful to use the transesophageal echo to guide passage of the pulmonary artery catheter.

Filling the balloon with 1 mL of sterile saline reveals a beautiful echogenic image, which can easily be followed through the atrium and ventricle into the pulmonary artery — quite a visual treat.

Caveat:

Some counsel against filling the balloon with liquid because of the possibility that it may become trapped by a faulty valve, thus rendering it impossible to fully deflate the balloon for catheter withdrawal

M Heath, New York, USA

Excessive waveform "fling"

It may be difficult to recognise the correct pulmonary artery diastolic or occlusion pressure or left atrial "a" and "v" waves because of excessive waveform harmonics ("fling" or "whip"). These waves develop especially when there is redundant tubing length or multiple stopcocks in the system.

Tip:

There are several manoeuvres that can provide sufficient damping to remove excessive fling and make the wave form more easily interpretable:

- Put a tiny bubble of air in the line. If that works:
- Take the bubble out of the line and replace it with one in the transducer dome. It won't get flushed away.
- Place a 1 mL syringe (preferably with a Luer lock) on the side port of the stopcock to which the catheter tubing is attached. "Break" the stopcock, i.e. turn the lever so that the stopcock is open to the syringe.
- Place a "Heplock" on the side port of the stopcock to which the catheter tubing is attached and turn the lever so that the stopcock is open to the device. The Heplock is a small Luer locked fitting with a rubber cap which is normally placed on an intravenous catheter to allow it to be flushed with heparinized saline and preserve venous access without the need for a running intravenous line. The advantage of this approach is that the cap can be pierced by a needle to allow fluid to aspirate back. Thus, the size of the air bubble can be adjusted to modulate the degree of damping required.

P Lawler, Middlesbrough, UK
R N Sladen, New York, USA

Insertion of a pulmonary artery catheter

Sometimes pulmonary artery occlusion ("wedge") is achieved only at the time of catheter insertion, and thereafter is difficult or impossible to achieve.

Tip:

Always monitor both central venous (CVP, or right atrial) and pulmonary artery (PA) pressures as you advance the catheter. [This does require that you use two transducers but it is worth the extra trouble]. Make sure both transducers are zeroed at the same level and have the same gain (amplification) on the monitor. Then, when the catheter wedges, you can see whether the CVP and the pulmonary artery occlusion pressure (PAOP) are identical.

If you note the relationship between CVP and PAOP when the catheter is initially placed, you can make an educated guess about the PAOP from the CVP should you not be able to subsequently achieve wedge.

For example, assume both CVP and PAOP read 22 mmHg at the time of flotation (even if the number was obtained when the catheter was not at the phlebostatic axis). Later the pulmonary artery catheter stops wedging, but the CVP reads 22 mmHg. It would be reasonable to assume that PAOP is 22 mmHg as well.

In another example, suppose the PAOP reads 22 and the CVP 15 mmHg (i.e. left heart failure). Later the pulmonary artery catheter stops wedging, but the CVP increases to 18 mmHg. In this case, it is reasonable to assume that the PAOP has increased as well.

There are two other reasons for observing both CVP and PA waveforms on the screen during initial flotation, both related to watching the CVP trace pattern.

Caveat:

If during flotation the CVP trace starts showing a right ventricular waveform the CVP or right atrial port has been pushed through the tricuspid valve. The pulmonary artery catheter may have coiled in the right ventricle, that is, it has had to be pushed a long way in to get into the pulmonary artery. Eschew coiled catheters! They get caught up in chordae or migrate. If the catheter is NOT coiled, this indicates a big right ventricle. This itself is not a good sign. It might be full of clots and/or you are more likely to get arrhythmias.

Caveat:

If the CVP or right atrial port is in the right ventricle, automatic calculations of cardiac performance will be wrong. For example, calculation of systemic vascular resistance (SVR) requires input of the CVP. If the computer uses the mean right ventricular pressure instead (usually a higher number), the calculated SVR will be artifactually low.

P Lawler, Middlesbrough, UK

Prevention of pulmonary haemorrhage from a pulmonary artery catheter

The most dreaded complication of pulmonary artery catheterization is pulmonary artery rupture and massive haemorrhage.

The major risk factors for this complication include:

- pulmonary hypertension (increased sheer stress)
- coagulopathy or anticoagulation (continuous haemorrhage)
- advanced age (more friable vessels)
- excessive advancement of the pulmonary artery catheter into small vessels

Caveats:

1. Advance the catheter beyond 15 cm only when the balloon is fully inflated with 1.5 mL air.

Do this exercise next time you are getting ready to float a pulmonary artery catheter. Inflate the balloon with 0.5 mL air. Nothing happens. Inflate the balloon with 1.0 mL air. The balloon partially inflates but does not project beyond the tip of the catheter (this predisposes to contact arrhythmias). Inflate the balloon with 1.5 mL air. It finally expands to its full rotundity. Floatation of the pulmonary artery catheter with a hypoinflated balloon will result in occlusion in a small, distal arterial branch. If someone subsequently inflates the balloon with 1.5 mL air, vessel rupture is possible.

2. Set limits for advancement of the catheter to achieve pulmonary artery occlusion.

For the right internal jugular approach in an average sized adult, this should be approximately 55 cm at the skin. Add 5 cm for the left internal jugular approach or for a large patient or dilated heart. From the femoral vein, occlusion should be achieved by 80 cm. Obeying these limits is probably the single most important means of prevention of distal catheterization, the most proximate cause of pulmonary artery rupture.

3. Always inflate the balloon slowly to achieve pulmonary artery occlusion.

If there is excessive resistance, or if an occlusion pressure tracing is achieved with less than 1.0 mL air, or if the pressure tracing starts to climb off the recording paper ("overwedge", due to occlusion of the catheter port by balloon compression) — you are out too far! Stop, pull back 2–3 cm, and try again.

4. When deflating the balloon, quickly remove the syringe to allow prompt balloon collapse

Slow balloon deflation by withdrawing air with the syringe may allow a partially inflated balloon to sweep the catheter out into a more distal position.

R N Sladen, New York, USA

Positive end-expiratory pressure and pulmonary artery wedging

If a pulmonary artery catheter is floated in patient on positive end-expiratory pressure (PEEP) the catheter could become "stranded". In this situation, the blood column between the catheter tip and the left atrium is discontinuous, and the PAOP is in fact the transmitted alveolar pressure.

Tip:

Increase PEEP during advancement of the pulmonary artery catheter from the pulmonary artery to the wedged position. This prevents "stranding".

P Lawler, Middlesbrough, UK

Unsure of pulmonary artery catheter position

Occasionally, it is difficult to determine whether a waveform that looks “wedged” is in fact the pulmonary artery occlusion pressure.

Tip:

Take two blood samples from the pulmonary artery port: one with the balloon deflated (i.e. a mixed venous sample) and inflated (wedged sample). If the wedged PO_2 exceeds the mixed venous PO_2 then the catheter truly is in the wedged position when the balloon is inflated. The PO_2 is higher because blood is being withdrawn from the pulmonary artery capillaries.

Caveat:

If the blood withdrawn from the wedged catheter looks arterial in colour, and the PO_2 is almost identical to the arterial PO_2, the catheter may be too far in. Blood is being sampled from the left atrium!

P Lawler, Middlesbrough, UK
R N Sladen, New York, USA

CHAPTER 5

VASCULAR CANNULATION

Positioning the patient

One of the most important causes of failed or difficult venous cannulation is inadequate light or improper patient position.

Tip:

Spend enough time getting the patient in the right position — a minute or two here will save many minutes of frustration for the operator and reduce the risk to the patient.

Pump the bed up to a reasonable working height (usually as high as it will go) to avoid bending your back. Then, if cannulation proves difficult and takes time you will not get backache!

Ensure you have a good light.

G R Park, Cambridge, UK

Finding the internal jugular vein

In many patients the internal jugular vein may be difficult to find, or may be collapsed due to hypovolaemia.

Tip:

There are a number of manoeuvres that can be tried in an attempt to make central extrathoracic veins bigger and easier to cannulate:

Put the head down and feet up (Trendelenburg position) — this should be used for all central cannulation to decrease the risk of entraining air and venous air embolism.

In patients on mechanical ventilation, try increasing PEEP, the I-E ratio, or the plateau pressure.

Caveat:

This does not work for the intrathoracic veins and may be dangerous in some patients. Press on the liver (i.e. induce hepatojugular reflux).

P Lawler, Middlesbrough, UK
M J Lindop, Cambridge, UK

Tip:

In a non-intubated patient who can cooperate, a forced Val Salva manoeuvre (forced expiration against a closed glottis) increases venous pressure and markedly distends the jugular vein. Ask the patient to "bear down". You will be surprised at how much this improves your success rate!

R N Sladen, New York, USA

Seeking the central vein

Most complications of venous cannulation are related to placement of a large bore needle in the wrong place — through the vein or pleura, or into an artery!

Tip:

ALWAYS use at least a 21-gauge needle to locate the vein — not just for internal jugular vein access, but also for subclavian and femoral cannulation. A smaller needle allows for better "feel" of the anatomy, including thick clavicles. Also, 21-gauge holes close much faster than 18-gauge holes, especially in arteries and pleura!

D MacGregor, Winston-Salem, North Carolina, USA

Turn the sound up!

Complications of venous cannulation may be heralded by arrhythmias or hypoxemia.

Tip:

- Turn the sound up on the ECG and pulse oximeter.
- When the guidewire is in the right ventricle there is commonly a salvo of ectopics, so you realise your wire is being advanced in the correct direction.
- It will tell you if arrhythmias are persistent.
- A sudden decrease in oxygen saturation or bradycardia may indicate hypoxaemia — which may be caused by a tension pneumothorax.

P Lawler, Middlesbrough, UK

Inadvertent arterial puncture

If you inadvertently puncture a large artery, the immediate reflex is to put pressure on the artery.

Tip:

Instead, quickly make another attempt at venous cannulation. The arterial bleeding will tamponade the vein and cause it to collapse — not only is the vein distorted, but the vein will be collapsed and compressed by the expanding haematoma. Once you have achieved venous access, or if you don't rapidly succeed, then compress the artery.

Caveat:

Don't try this on someone who is anticoagulated or who has a coagulopathy!

Also, if a non-intubated patient develops a large neck haematoma, avoid the temptation to try to cannulate the opposite side of the neck. Bilateral haematomas can compromize the airway! Look for an alternative site away from the neck, e.g. subclavian or femoral vein.

P Lawler, Middlesborough, UK
R N Sladen, New York, USA

Femoral vein cannulation

Occasionally it may be difficult to access the femoral vein.

Tip:

Remember "VAN" (**v**ein, **a**rtery, **n**erve). The femoral vein is always just medial to the femoral artery. Palpate the femoral artery and then make your approach just medial to it.

Put a sandbag under the buttock on the same side. This makes the leg rotate externally, giving easier access to the femoral vein.

S Ridley, Norwich, UK
R N Sladen, New York

Internal jugular cannulation

Occasionally there may be difficulty defining the anatomy of the sternomastoid triangle (i.e. the triangle made by the sternal and clavicular heads, and the clavicle.)

Tip:

Gently palpate the carotid artery. The internal jugular vein lies just lateral to the pulse. Aim your needle just lateral and pointing to the nipple.

J Thompson, Scunthorpe, UK

Caveat:

Don't press too hard on the carotid artery or you will compress the vein as well.

M J Lindop, Cambridge, UK

Tip:

Put your finger tip in the suprasternal notch. You should be able to define this even in obese patients. Then, gently slide your finger laterally above the clavicle. The next "valley" your finger falls into is the sternomastoid triangle. Go to the apex and aim your finder needle along the lateral edge, in the direction of the ipsilateral nipple.

R N Sladen, New York, USA

Subclavian vein cannulation

Occasionally a venous catheter placed into the subclavian vein goes upwards into the internal jugular vein, rather than downwards into the superior vena cava.

Tip:

To recognise when a subclavian central line has gone into the jugular system, simply attach a pressure monitoring line to the distal lumen port. Observe the pressure trace whilst gently compressing the neck. If the tip lies within the jugular system, the waveform will flatten with neck compression. The line can now be repositioned until the waveform is unaffected by neck compression.

J Gannon, Wirral, UK

For subclavian vein cannulation, does it matter if one uses the left or right side?

Tip:

Choose the left side in preference. The catheter threads move easily because it follows the natural curve of the innominate vein into the superior vena cava. From the right side, it has to make a sharp turn.

M J Lindop, Cambridge, UK

There are a number of suggestions that exist for correct positioning of the patient for the insertion of a subclavian catheter via the supraclavicular or infraclavicular approach:

- Place a pillow between the shoulder blades
- Ask an assistant to pull the arm down (caudally)
- Push the head to the opposite side

Caveat:

- When a pillow is placed between the shoulder blades, the shoulders fall back and compress the vein between the clavicle and the first rib
- When the arm is pulled down the vein is stretched and made smaller
- Pushing the head to the opposite side also stretches the vein

Tip:

The best position is a relaxed one: small pillow under head, arm lying gently by the side.

P Lawler, Middlesbrough, UK

External jugular vein cannulation

External jugular cannulation often looks tempting because the vein is distended and easily visible. To one's chagrin, success is not so easily attained. During insertion, the vein collapses or rolls away and a large haematoma is the fruit of one's labours.

Tip:

External jugular cannulation is most reliably accomplished using the Seldinger technique (needle, guidewire, catheter) or catheter over the needle technique.

Before you start, bend the needle or intravenous catheter slightly so that it does not catch on the jaw, and make sure you can thread the catheter past the bend. Turn the patient's head away from you, tamponade the vein distally with your left index finger, and use your left thumb to put traction on the skin.

When you are ready, make a quick, precise stab into the vessel and insert the catheter. If you meet resistance to insertion of the guidewire or catheter, have an assistant abduct the arm, and, if necessary pull it anteriorly over the chest. This will open the space at the clavicle and the wire and catheter will advance with ease.

D B Coursin, Madison, Wisconsin, USA

Pulmonary artery cannulation via the external jugular vein

If the patient has a severe coagulopathy there may be reluctance to cannulate the internal jugular or subclavian veins or there may be a reason to avoid the femoral route.

Tip:

I have had occasional success cannulating the external jugular vein for pulmonary artery catheterization. The trick here is to secure the external jugular vein with the pulmonary artery introducer in the usual manner — but do not advance the introducer beyond the "bend" of the external jugular vein as it joins the subclavian vein. Attempts to do so will either meet with obstruction or even rupture the vein. Instead, insert the introducer part way, then let the much more malleable pulmonary artery catheter itself negotiate the junction of the external jugular and subclavian veins, and make the sharp bend into the central circulation.

D B Coursin, Madison, Wisconsin, USA

The Seldinger technique

The most commonly used method to access the central venous circulation is the Seldinger technique. This relies on initial needle access to the vein, followed by placement of a malleable guidewire to secure access. Once the needle is removed, catheters, dilators, and/or introducers can be passed over the guidewire. Occasionally, difficulty is encountered in threading the guidewire through the needle.

Tip:

If the standard guidewire does not thread easily consider a Bentsen cerebral guidewire, used in angiography. It has a very fine and slippery end, which allows circumnavigation of difficult vessel angles. It is expensive, but usually saves the day.

D W Ryan, Newcastle-upon-Tyne, UK

Tip:

Always have the guidewire in your field of vision when performing central venous cannulation. Once the vein is perforated and free blood is aspirated it is important not to take your eye off the needle. If you start looking for the guidewire at this point, the needle tip will move, probably out of the vein.

S Ridley, Norwich, UK

Tip:

When you remove the guidewire from the introducer, re-sheath it in the plastic cover in which it came. This not only preserves the J-shaped tip in the case of reuse, but also prevents spraying droplets of blood around the ICU during disposal.

J O'Hanlon, Belfast, UK

When placing a central line in the internal jugular or subclavian vein, it is imperative to ensure that the guide wire has not inadvertently been placed into the carotid or subclavian artery.

Tip:

If one has transthoracic or transesophageal echocardiography in place or available, I use the image to corroborate correct placement. During insertion, the guide wire should be easily seen in the superior vena cava and/or right atrium. To distinguish the guide wire from a previously placed pacing lead or other central line, I position the wire so that the "J" hook at the end is caught in cross section by the echo plane. One then sees two separate "dots". By spinning the guide wire one dot is made to "dance" around the other, providing unmistakable confirmation of correct placement.

M Heath, New York, USA

When performing a central venous catheter placement using the Seldinger technique, there is always the possibility of exiting the vessel and causing a mediastinal haematoma.

Tip:

Make sure that the guidewire slides in and out with ease as you slide the catheter in. This avoids or limits this complication.

D B Coursin, Madison, Wisconsin, USA

Bleeding from line sites

Troublesome bleeding may occur from line sites both in the situation where the line remains *in situ* and is a loose fit, or after line removal. The bleeding may be arterial or venous. The problem may result from coagulation abnormality, movement of the line in and out of its puncture site, or too large an initial incision for the line.

Tip:

After correction of coagulation factors, local pressure, application of haemostatic cellulose (Surgicell) consider the following:

- Use a very fine (5.0/6.0) nylon vascular suture (from the operating theatre), and a pair of suitable needle holders.
- Put a purse string suture round a line *in situ*, or in the case of lines being removed put sutures across the insertion site. Such manoeuvres stabilise blood clot and will usually stop the bleeding.

Caveat:

Do not be tempted to try the same with a typical large diameter silk anchoring suture, as this makes large holes and will only make the problems worse.

A R Bodenham, Leeds, UK

Suturing in an introducer

After placement of a large introducer for central venous monitoring or pulmonary artery catheterization, security and local haemostasis are essential.

Tip:

Once the introducer has been inserted, a simple secure, hemostatic suture can be placed as follows:

1. Use a straight needle and 3-0 silk or the suture provided in the kit.
2. Enter the skin at "1 o'clock" relative to the introducer as you look down at it from the head of the patient.
3. Tunnel subcutaneously in a "U" around the introducer and exit the skin at "11 o'clock". Voila! — you have a "purse string" suture.
4. Tie down directly on to the skin, twice. The suture is much easier to handle if you keep it on full stretch and make your knots with some tension on the suture. Make your knots firm but not too tight — you want hemostasis, not skin necrosis!
5. Without cutting the suture, take the needle and thread it through the "eye" of the introducer, and tie down directly on to it, twice, as above. Now cut the redundant suture with the blade provided in the kit.

6. Test the security of your tie by gently tugging on the introducer. It should be fixed in place. If your suture is too lax, cut and start over!

When you get slick, this should take you less than thirty seconds!

R N Sladen, New York, USA

Arterial cannulation

Radial artery catheterization

Radial artery catheterization is one of the most common procedures in the ICU but occasionally can cause considerable frustration and time delay, not to mention anguish for the patient.

Tip:

Success in radial artery catheterization can be markedly improved by correct positioning of the wrist and hand.

1. "Cock" the wrist by taping the hand and arm to a flat armboard and placing a small rolled towel or bandage under the wrist. Then gently but firmly hyperextend and tape the thumb down so that the skin over the radial artery is pulled taut.
2. Infiltrate the skin over the radial artery with local anaesthetic (do this even in an unconscious patient — it helps prevent arterial spasm) and rub well to spread it out and allow easy palpation of the pulse.
3. Plug the catheter cover into the back of the catheter so you have a longer reservoir in which to observe blood pulsation.

4. Gently palpate the artery with the fingers of your left (or non dominant) hand, and use as flat an approach as possible (i.e. a narrow angle between catheter and skin) to maximize the contact area between needle and artery.
5. Advance slowly but continuously toward the pulse felt by your fingers. If you hit bone, pull back and flatten out the catheter.
6. Successful cannulation is evidenced by pulsatile backflow of bright red blood into the catheter and reservoir. Advance the catheter over the needle, making sure that backflow continues.
7. If the backflow stops at any stage, pull the catheter back onto its original position on the needle, then slowly withdraw the catheter and needle until the backflow reappears, then readvance the catheter over the needle.
8. If you get a "flash" of backflow with your first advance, it means you have gone through the artery. This is usually not a problem. Follow step 7 above!

It is not uncommon to get a flashback, but then not be able to advance the catheter. This may be due to an intimal flap, kinking or stenosis.

Tip:

Passing a guidewire (a narrow gauge French size 35 may be required) may allow the catheter to be advanced. For this reason, it is always wise to provide a sterile work area and wear sterile gloves when a difficult cannulation is anticipated. Alternatively, kits are available with an integrated guidewire although the "feel" for cannulation is less sensitive.

It is not necessary to suture the arterial catheter in place if you use tincture of benzoin and pink tape!

When you tape the catheter in place, be sure to make a loop of the tubing between the thumb and forefinger, and then back on to the wrist. That way, if someone inadvertently pulls on the tubing, there is less chance of the catheter being immediately pulled back or out.

R N Sladen, New York, USA

Inadvertent carotid artery cannulation

Inadvertent carotid artery cannulation is a startling and potentially catastrophic complication, depending on the size of introducer or catheter inserted. However, there are ways to stay out of more trouble!

Tip:

If the patient has a severe coagulopathy, correct it before removing the catheter.

If the patient has only a small disturbance of clotting or none, remove the catheter as soon as possible.

Do NOT use it for:

- monitoring
- taking blood samples
- infusing drugs

Increased manipulation of the line increases the risk of cerebral infarction.

Do not attach a three-way tap to it — this risks inadvertent injection of a drug

Put a large label on it warning that it is an arterial line, until it is removed.

G R Park, Cambridge, UK

Impalpable arteries

Oedematous arms, legs and feet can make determining the location of arteries difficult.

Tip:

Place a Doppler probe above expected site and manoeuvre it until the pulsatile flow signal is at its loudest. Advance the arterial catheter toward the probe in the usual way using the signal to determine placement. The artery can usually be located without difficulty.

D W Ryan, Newcastle-upon-Tyne, UK

Anterograde radial artery cannulation

Difficulty may be encountered in placing a radial artery catheter in a site previously cannulated. There may be partial obstruction of the radial artery proximal to the previous cannulation site by clot or an intimal flap. During retrograde cannulation blood flows freely, but the catheter cannot be advanced beyond the obstruction.

Tip:

Consider anterograde cannulation. Directing the catheter towards thumb is often successful, while not compromising palmar arch flow.

Caveat:

Ensure that the nursing staff know that the catheter has been inserted in the "wrong" direction, so that they don't try to reposition it, thinking that it must be kinked!

N Cohen, San Francisco, California, USA

Too much "fling" in the arterial pressure tracing

Systolic and diastolic pressures may be artifactually too high and too low if harmonic resonant waves are set up in an underdamped system. This is especially likely to occur with long tubing and several stopcocks.

Tip:

Put a tiny air bubble in the transducer top to dampen the frequency response.

Caveat:

If you put in too much air, you'll get an overdamped tracing, with artifactually low systolic pressure. However, the mean arterial pressure will still generally be representative.

P Lawler, Middlesbrough, UK

Axillary artery cannulation

Patients who have been in the ICU for a long time often become increasingly difficult to cannulate.

Tip:

Consider axillary artery cannulation. Perform it as if you were doing an axillary block, but cannulate the artery instead! This is more successful in the patient who does not move his/her arm too much.

Caveat:

Make sure you use a catheter that is of sufficient length.

P B Lumb, Albany, New York, USA

Is your system damping optimal?

Overdamping causes systolic to underread and diastolic to overread: underdamping causes the systolic to overread and the diastolic to underread

Tip:

- Pump the pressure infusor to >300 mmHg
- "Fast flush" the transducer (pull the "tail", and then let go)
- Wait two seconds and then freeze the screen
- Look at the trace:
  - no overshoot means overdamped
  - two overshoots is just right
  - three or more means the system is resonating

P Lawler, Middlesbrough, UK

Not sure if you are in an artery when doing a single stab for a blood gas?

Tip:

Use a Butterfly® cannula. Intermittent (or even infusion) Butterfly® needles have a long, flexible (i.e. compliant) length of tubing between the needle and injection port or Luer lock. When exploring for your blood gas, the blood not only flashes back, but can be seen to pulsate. It is the pulsation that tells you you are in the artery, not the colour of blood. The needle is also very short bevel, which means you tend not to go through the vessel and out the other side. Once in the vessel, you can attach a syringe to the bung or Luer lock and take the blood sample. You can even leave the Butterfly® in the artery for an hour or two.

P Lawler, Middlesbrough, UK

Test for palmar collateral circulation

In patients with compromized peripheral circulation, it may be reassuring to confirm that there is adequate anastomotic circulation when you obstruct the radial artery with a cannula.

Traditionally, the Allen's test has been advocated: the patient opens and closes a fist rapidly three or four times while you occlude both radial and ulnar arteries. Then, the patient opens his hand and you release ulnar compression. A "flush" passing down the blanched hand within five seconds is a normal response which indicates patency of the ulnar artery and palmar collateral circulation.

Unfortunately, a normal Allen test does not guarantee distal compromise by a radial artery catheter, and the test is not feasible in sedated ICU patients.

Tip:

Pulse oximeters are exquisitely sensitive pulse detecting devices. Put a pulse oximeter probe on a finger and occlude the artery with your thumb: if there is no ulnar circulation you will lose the pulse wave.

P Lawler, Middlesbrough, UK

CHAPTER 6

INOTROPES

Multiple drug infusions

It is convenient to provide multiple drug infusions vis a single central venous catheter. However, when dose changes are made with slow infusion rates, there may be considerable delay before the new rate is effective because of dead space in the tubing. Then, when the drug finally reaches the central circulation, there may be an abrupt increase in concentration.

Caveat:

Always provide a "carrier" solution running at a reasonable rate, e.g. 50 mL/h, into which drug infusions are piggy-backed. This will ensure timely and smooth alterations in delivered concentration when you adjust the drug infusion dose.

R N Sladen, New York, USA

Haemodynamically unstable patients who are dependent on potent inotropic and vasopressor drugs can suffer a substantial decrease in blood pressure and cardiac output when the infusions are disrupted by the necessity to change syringe drivers. All syringe drivers have a lag time before they are up to speed when they are switched on, some more than others, while the drive mechanism takes up slack in the drive system and pressurizes the syringe. Piggy-backing a replacement syringe can negate the time taken to change syringes by the nursing staff, but does not overcome the inherent syringe lag time.

Tip:

The following method overcomes both the nursing delay and the syringe driver lag time in changing syringes and should minimize any haemodynamic perturbations:

1. Connect a second syringe via a 3-way stopcock to the side port of a 3-way stopcock which is used to connect the original syringe to the venous line.
2. Start the second syringe at the correct rate before the primary syringe is finished, but allow it to vent to atmosphere via the side arm of its own 3-way stopcock.
3. After 15 minutes or the time taken for this syringe to reach the correct speed according to the manufacturer's instruction booklet, swiftly switch the two 3-way stopcocks to connect the second syringe to the patient's venous line and then disconnect the original syringe and re-charge it.

P V Woodsford, Glamorgan, Wales

Inotropes not working

Occasionally it appears as if a patient is receiving no benefit from an inotropic agent or vasopressor.

Tip:

Check that it is being delivered to the patient!

Is the syringe pump working? Is the central venous line kinked, obstructed or displaced?

K E Gunning, Cambridge, UK

Doses

Calculation of drug infusion rates in μg/kg/min can be time consuming.

Tip:

Dilute the equivalent of the inotropic agent in mg of three times the patient body weight in kg in 50 mL fluid. Then, each 1 mL/h then provides 1 μg/kg/min.

For example, for an 80 kg patient dilute 240 mg dopamine in 50 mL. Then, 3 mL/h would provide 3 μg/kg/min.

S Ridley, Norwich, UK

Tip:

Here is a simple bedside method of calculating drug infusion rates in μg/kg/min. Most times, you still do need a calculator!

- Check the drug concentration, and correct to 1000 mL.
- The number of mg/1000 mL = μg/mL.
- Divide this by the patient's weight in kg.
- Multiply this by the infusion rate and divide by 60.

For example, suppose an 80 kg man has dopamine (400 mg in 250 mL) running at 6 mL/h.

400 mg/250 mL = 1600 mg/1000 mL = 1600 μg/mL.

Then, 1600/80 × 6/60 = 2 μg/kg/min.

R N Sladen, New York, USA

Starting inodilators

Inodilators (e.g. dobutamine, dopexamine, milrinone) are inotropic agents with potent vasodilator effects. Starting them in a patient who is hypovolemic can result in abrupt hypotension.

Caveat:

Ensure that the patient is adequately fluid resuscitated before starting an inodilator, and be prepared to administer fluids rapidly once the infusion begins.

M L Pepperman, Leicester, UK

Use of sodium nitroprusside

Administration of a potent vasodilator such as sodium nitroprusside, especially in a hypovolaemic patient, can be associated with marked swings in blood pressure. For example, starting too fast results in acute hypotension. Then, switching the infusion off results in rebound hypertension and overshoot.

Caveat:

Use the principle of "masterly underreaction". Make small adjustments in dose rate early, rather than large adjustments late!

R N Sladen, New York, USA

CHAPTER 7

NEUROLOGICAL SYSTEM

Unexpected coma

Occasionally, a patient may become unexpectedly unresponsive or unconscious.

Tip:

Study the drug chart carefully. Remember, short-acting sedative and analgesic drugs may be long-acting in the critically ill. Use the antagonists naloxone and flumazenil — unless there is a contraindication such as raised intracranial pressure or the risk of fits.

G R Park, Cambridge, UK

Treatment of elevated intracranial pressure

After severe head injury, intracranial pressure may be elevated. Maintenance of adequate cerebral perfusion pressure (i.e. mean arterial pressure minus intracranial pressure) is essential.

Tip:

A simple way of testing for adequate cerebral perfusion is to increase the mean arterial pressure with a small dose of a vasoconstrictor such as phenylpehrine.

If intracranial pressure decreases, it means that a higher dose is required to reduce reflex cerebral vasodilatation.

Take steps to increase the patient's mean arterial pressure during further management.

B Matta, Cambridge, UK

Guillain-Barré syndrome and other polyneuropathies

Close assessment of patients with new onset polyneuropathy is essential to determine their requirement for ICU admission.

Tip:

Ask the patient to perform peak flow measurements every hour

See if they can:

- Lift their arms and grasp the peak flow meter (arm and hand strength and co-ordination)
- Purse their lips around the meter (co-ordination of facial muscle, and lips)

You can then monitor peak expiratory flow rate (PEFR), arm weakness, and facial weakness simultaneously.

If you are still not sure of their abilty to protect their airway, ask the patient to swallow a glass of water.

Can they:

- Lift the glass?
- Purse their lips?
- Swallow?
- Protect their airway? (does the water come out of their nose, and does it make them cough?)
- Is the cough adequate?

If the answer to any of these questions is "No", admit the patient to the ICU for airway control and possible mechanical ventilation.

Arterial blood gases are of no help in deciding that the patient needs respiratory support: blood gases FOLLOW the clinical condition rather than precede it.

P Lawler, Middlesbrough, UK

Tracheal intubation

Caveat:

- Patients are ALWAYS dehydrated (can't, don't or won't swallow, sweat too much).
- Patients often have a dysautonomia:

  They cannot increase their heart rate or vasoconstrict appropriately in response to vasodilatation or hypovolemia. Hypotension follows.
- There is a constant potential for sudden vagal dominance and severe bradycardia.

Tip:

- Rehydrate — give the patient 1–2 litres of intravenous fluid while you get your equipment ready.
- Make sure that both the ECG and pulse oximeter provide audible pulse monitoring during laryngoscopy and intubation.
- Give intravenous atropine before tracheal intubation, or have it ready to administer at the first signs of bradycardia.

P Lawler, Middlesbrough, UK

Epidural haematoma

Epidural haematoma is a rare but devastating complication of epidural catheters. Although it may occur in the non-anticoagulated patient, the risk is increased with the use of anticoagulation. Administration of fibrinolytic agents (e.g. urokinase) is an absolute contraindication to epidural catheter placement.

Tip:

Not only is there a risk of this complication at insertion of the catheter, but also when it is removed. To reduce the risk of an epidural haematoma and consequent neurological injury do not remove the catheter until eight–twelve hours after heparin and the PTT has corrected to normal.

Caveat:

Low molecular weight heparin (e.g. danaparin) is being used more and more because of its convenient twice a day dosage and the decreased risk of heparin-associated thrombocytopenia.

However, its anticoagulant effect cannot be monitored by the PTT but requires a special assay (activated factor X level).

Tip:

In patients on low molecular weight heparin do not remove the epidural catheter until eight to twelve hours have passed since the last dose AND don't redose for two hours after removal of the catheter.

G R Park, Cambridge, UK

CHAPTER 8

MISCELLANEOUS TIPS ABOUT DRUGS

There are many tips and caveats about drugs. Some you will find in other chapters, others in textbooks of pharmacology (see, for example, *Drug Prescribing in Anaesthesia and Intensive Care*, H G Paw and G R Park, Greenwich Medical Media Ltd, *Handbook of Drugs in Intensive Care*, H G Paw and G R Park or *Algorithms for Rational Prescribing in the Critically Ill*, N Evans and G R Park, Blackwell Healthcare Publication), *Pharmacology in the Critically Ill*, Eds. G R Park and M P Shelly, BMJ Publications Ltd.

Verapamil

Verapamil is the calcium channel blocker with the most potent effect on blocking atrioventricular conduction, and is very effective in the treatment of supraventricular tachycardia (SVT), especially atrial tachycardia. However, it also dilates peripheral blood vessels which may cause unwanted hypotension during treatment in a patient whose blood pressure may already be lowered by the arrhythmia.

Tip:

Give 1 gram (10 mL) calcium chloride intravenously before dosing verapamil. This opposes its peripheral vasodilatatory effect, but not its anti-arrhythmic effect.

P Lawler, Middlesbrough, UK

Tip:

An alternative is to administer 50–200 μg intravenous phenylephrine before verapamil. Not only will this prevent or counteract the vasodilator effect of verapamil, but the ensuing increase in blood pressure and vagal tone may enhance the probability of converting the SVT back to sinus rhythm.

R N Sladen, New York, USA

Drug Interactions

Cisapride, Fluconazole and Erythromycin*

Cisapride (10 mg 8 hourly via NGT) is an effective agent to enhance gastric emptying.

*Cisapride has been withdrawn in the UK and USA because of the risk of potentially fatal arrythmias.

Caveat:

The combination of cisapride with fluconazole or erythromycin can prolong the QT interval.

P Lawler, Middlesbrough, UK

Diltiazem and Digoxin

Diltiazem by intravenous infusion is a useful "slowing" agent to control the ventricular response during rapid atrial fibrillation while the patient is being loaded with digoxin.

Caveat:

Diltiazem impairs renal elimination of digoxin, and plasma digoxin levels should be closely monitored.

Diltiazem and Cyclosporin A

There is now convincing evidence that perioperative administration of diltiazem can protect the transplanted kidney against the nephrotoxic effects of cyclosporin A.

Caveat:

Diltiazem inhibits cyclosporin metabolism and decreases its elimination by about one third. Therefore, administration of standard doses of cyclosporin A may result in "toxic" blood levels.

However, diltiazem still protects the kidney in this situation and the net effect is a decreased incidence of rejection. A one third reduction of the dose of cyclosporin A can also realise a substantial cost savings for long term immunosuppressive therapy.

About drugs

In the ICU, there is always a risk of confusion and mistakes in drug ordering — in both name and dosage. Often, the original indication for a drug becomes obscure, as more and more drugs are "layered on", sometimes to treat side effects caused by the previous one!

Tip:

1. Write orders in the drug chart in clear block capitals.
2. Always try and stop an existing drug rather than start a new one.

   e.g. if the systemic vascular resistance (SVR) is too high, stop dopamine before starting sodium nitroprusside!
3. When ordering antibiotics, give their indication and a date to stop or review them. It makes later decisions about them easier.

Date	Time	Antibiotic/ dose	Indication	Date to stop or review

G R Park, Cambridge, UK

Potassium and the β receptor

The interaction between beta-adrenergic state and potassium flux is not widely known. Normally, the intracellular concentration of potassium (160 mEq/L) is about 40 times as great as the extracellular concentration (4 mEq/L). Potassium is pumped into the cell against its concentration gradient by a sodium-potassium ATPase pump, which is closely regulated by beta-adrenergic tone.

Beta-adrenergic stimulation increases potassium flux into the cell, whereas beta-blockade inhibits its uptake.

Tip:

In the emergency treatment of a patient with acute hyperkalemia, administration of a β-agonist can decrease serum potassium levels.

Examples include intravenous dobutamine or aerosol administration of a bronchodilator such as terbutaline, salbutamol or albuterol.

Caveat:

High doses of a β-blocker (including labetolol) in a patient in renal failure could exacerbate hyperkalemia.

R N Sladen, New York, USA

Propofol and nutritional intake

Propofol is highly lipid soluble and is delivered in a 10% fat emulsion — the same fat emulsion that is used in total parenteral nutrition. Continuous sedation with propofol can therefore contribute a substantial amount of fat calories.

Caveat:

Deduct the fat calories provided by propofol infusion when calculating parenteral or enteral nutritional intake.

For example, if an 80 kg patient is receiving propofol at 50 μg/kg/min, the total amount of propofol delivered per hour would be (0.050 × 80 × 60) = 240 mg. The concentration of propofol is 10 mg/mL, so the volume of 10% fat emulsion is 24 mL/hr or close to 600 mL/day. With 10% fat emulsion, 1 mL provides 1 kcal.

In other words, this patient would be receiving 600 kcal/day day of fat calories, and the total nutritional intake should be adjusted accordingly.

In some parts of the world 2% propofol is available, which provides 0.5 kcal/mL fat emulsion. Calculations should be adjusted accordingly.

R N Sladen, New York, USA

CHAPTER 9

INFECTION

Gentamicin

Gentamicin is cheap, and kills bacteria rapidly. Virtually 100% of Gram-negative bacteria infecting patients recently admitted to UK ICUs remain gentamicin sensitive. Also, as far as I am aware, one day of gentamicin therapy is not likely to cause nephro- or oto-toxicity.

Tip:

In an acutely septic, newly admitted patient, consider adding a single dose of gentamicin (5–7 mg/kg) overnight until the preliminary results of cultures are available the following day. The antibiotic regimen can then be modified according to what has grown.

This strategy can also be useful for patients who have been on the ICU longer, but only in units who know they have low rates of gentamicin resistance.

M Farrington, Cambridge, UK

About antibiotics

The number of antibiotics an ICU patient is receiving tends towards the number of specialist teams who have seen them, plus one.

Caveat:

Every day, for every antibiotic, you should ask "Why is this patient being given this dangerous drug?"

The "Performance Indicator" for a successful daily microbiology ICU round should be to stop more antibiotics than you start!

M Farrington, Cambridge, UK

Otitis media

The middle ear drains when the body is upright. Critically ill patients are supine for long times. Because the ear cannot drain, secretions build up. These can then become infected by haematogenous spread or by bacteria getting access from the Eustachian tube. Not only is it a source of infection it is very painful.

Tip:

As part of an infection screen, always look in the ears.

G R Park, Cambridge, UK

Acute sinusitis

Patients with nasal tubes (endotracheal tubes, nasogastric tubes or silastic feeding tubes) may develop nosocomial (usually Gram-negative) infection of their facial sinuses within 48 hours of admission to the ICU. These frequently become a reservoir for direct or haematogenous spread to other organs, especially the lungs.

Tip:

Change nasotracheal tubes to the oral route within 48 hours of placement.

In a patient on long term nasogatric or nasojejunal feeding with recurrent fevers, consider performing a percutaneous endoscopic gastrostomy (PEG) to allow removal of the catheters from the nose. If a jejunal tube is necessary it can be passed via the gastrostomy.

Always consider acute sinusitis in the differential diagnosis of new onset, persistent or recurrent fever and/or infection in ICU patients. Clinical examination, X-rays or ultimately, even CT scanning may be required to confirm the diagnosis.

R N Sladen, New York, USA

Use of aseptic technique for procedures

Our hospital charges a great deal for every blood culture, complete blood count, differential count, and antibiotic. The one thing our hospital does NOT charge extra for is sterility!

Caveat:

We can use all the gowns, gloves, masks, sterile towels, etc. that we want to put in a central line, pulmonary artery catheter, arterial catheter, or chest tube. Prevention of even a single procedure-related infection by creating wide sterile fields saves the hospital far more money than the cost of sterile acoutrements and provides an infinite benefit to cost ratio. Also, you're fooling no-one but yourself if you think you can always prevent a guidewire from hitting your forearm during insertion of a catheter by the Seldinger technique. Put a gown on!

P B Lumb, Albany, New York, USA

CHAPTER 10

AGITATION, CONFUSION AND SEDATION

ICU-induced disorientation

Spatio-temporal disorientation is extremely common in ICU patients. This is caused by continuous physical and psychological discomfort, bright light, noise, with very little distinction between night and day.

Tip:

Here are a few tips to keep your patients more assured and oriented, and less confused and alienated:

- Talk to your patient each day. Hold their hand, look into their eyes and tell them that they are going to be OK.
- Try saying (if you believe it): "We're going to get you out of here. We're going to get you home". At least the patient will start to think that you are on the same side!
- If you don't think that they are going to make it, try saying "We're going to do everything we can to help you, and make you comfortable".
- Tell your patient what time of day it is, the date, where they are and (gently) what is happening to them. Do this each time you visit them.
- Post a clock and calendar prominently on the wall, where the patient can see them.
- Set up a strict daily schedule for meals, visiting hours, physical therapy and occupational therapy. Write up a schedule and post it on the wall so everyone working with the patient can see it.
- Prescribe a nighttime hypnotic. The tried and trusted combination of chloral hydrate and diphenhydramine still works well! But whatever you use, give it early in the evening. If the nurse is asking you for something for the patient at one o'clock in the morning, chances are they're going to have a pretty good lie-in the next day. So much for the ventilatory wean or physical therapy!

- Reduce stimulation at night! Eyeshades (the type they provide you with when you travel business class), and soft music played through headphones can work wonders.
- Don't forget the option of early, elective tracheostomy in the patient who is agitated and difficult to wean from the ventilator. It can make an enormous difference to their sense of comfort and interaction with their environment, and really give a boost to the ventilator wean.

R N Sladen, New York, USA

Administering sedative drugs

Bolus vs infusion

It is important to assess both the need and method of administration of sedative drugs.

Tip:

Give a bolus dose of a drug and ensure it has the desired effect. The time the drug acts for can also be noted. If it is a long time carry on with bolus doses. If it is short consider an infusion. Reassess the need for the infusion each day.

G R Park, Cambridge, UK

Accumulation of sedative drugs

Sedative drugs accumulate.

Tip:

Patients need more at the onset, following intubation and mechanical ventilation, but the infusion levels can often be reduced within a few hours to very modest doses. In general, the best dose of sedation is that with which the patient can tell you that they're comfortable.

M Singer, London, UK

Caveat:

It is very easy to start an infusion of a sedative or analgesic drug but much more difficult to stop. Infusions give large quantities of drugs each day. If the patient cannot eliminate them then they will accumulate resulting in coma.

Tip:

Unless the patient is awake or stopping the drug risks harm to the patient, stop all infusions daily. If the patient wakes up quickly and still has discomfort restart the infusion. If they take several hours to recover use a reduced dose or use intermittent bolus doses. Finally, if there is prolonged recovery use another drug.

G R Park, Cambridge, UK

Sedation scores

The level of sedation needs to be recorded frequently, like heart rate and blood pressure. Which score you use is not important. Use that one that suits your practice. The Addenbrooke's score is shown below, for reference.

The Addenbrooke's Sedation Score:

Agitated
Awake

Responds to spoken word
Responds to gentle shaking
Responds to tracheal suction*
No response to tracheal suction*
Paralysed/Asleep**
Pain Y/N
Comfortable on ventilator Y/N

* used instead of a painful stimulus
** sedation not assessed

This score (strictly a scale) is usually completed each hour during the acute period of illness.

G R Park, Cambridge, UK

Tip:

Use a sedation score to assess sedation! It doesn't matter which one you use, as long as you are consistent in its use.

A sedation score has at least three immediate benefits:

- Doctors and nurses start to talk the same language!
- The sedation score can be incorporated into the ICU flow sheet so that you can look back and appreciate the patient's level of sedation over the previous several hours.
- The sedation score may be used as a uniformly understood end-point for titration of drugs, for example, "Infuse midazolam to achieve a sedation score of 4".

The Ramsay Scale is an easy scoring system to remember. Its been around for more than twenty years, and it's dead simple.

1. agitation, always to be avoided.
2. calm and awake (as you were at the beginning of this chapter).
3. drowsy (as you are feeling when you read this!).

Scores of 4, 5 and 6 imply varying degrees of sleep:

4. the patient is asleep, but easily arousable.
5. the patient is asleep, but arousable with difficulty.
6. the patient is asleep, but unarousable.

Don't forget to indicate neuromuscular blockade by a "P" to remind everyone that muscle relaxants have no sedative, analgesic or amnesic action!

R N Sladen, New York, USA

Monitoring of neuromuscular blockade

When neuromuscular blockers are given it is first essential to ensure that the patient is deeply sedated and unarousable (e.g. Ramsay score 6). Then, especially when continuous infusion is used, it is essential to monitor the depth of neuromuscular blockade to avoid overdose, accumulation and delayed emergence. This is best achieved by dosing to preserve at least one twitch in the train of four.

Tip:

When you monitor a patient receiving neuromuscular blockade with a nerve stimulator using the train-of-four technique, don't just observe the fingers for twitch. Gently hold the patient's hand. You will be able to much more precisely determine the degree of fade and the number of twitches present by feel.

R N Sladen, New York, USA

Temperature measurement

There are differences in temperature between different sites in the body.

> **Caveat:**
>
> The pulmonary artery temperature is commonly measured and recorded when a pulmonary artery catheter is in place. Once it is removed the axillary temperature may be recorded, showing a false reduction in temperature.
>
> If the reverse occurs then an unexplained, false fever may occur.
>
> *G R Park, Cambridge, UK*

Tips on shivering after operation

Shivering occurs after cardiac surgery, major vascular surgery or any procedure in which patients develop intraoperative hypothermia.

At the end of hypothermic cardiopulmonary bypass, the central core is rewarmed to 37°C, but muscle and fat remain cold. After separation from cardiopulmonary bypass, heat redistributes itself from the warm core to the cold periphery, and the central temperature decreases ("afterdrop"). In the ICU, shivering begins as anaesthesia wears off and the hypothalamus responds to the decreased central temperature.

> **Caveat:**
>
> Shivering can dramatically increase central venous and pulmonary artery pressures. But the increase is only apparent. Shivering increases intrapleural pressure, which is transmitted into the intravascular space and reflected as spuriously high cardiac filling pressures.

Tip:

In a sedated, ventilated patient, administration of muscle relaxant can be used to abolish shivering and reveal the true hydrostatic pressures. Watch out — they could be pretty low!

Caveat:

Shivering markedly increases carbon dioxide production and mechanically ventilated patients may become acutely hypercarbic unless minute ventilation is increased or shivering treated.

Tip:

With the exception of patients with severe obstructive lung disease, capnometry is a sensitive and accurate guide to ventilatory requirement during shivering.

Caveat:

The central temperature or threshold for the onset of shivering is dependent on skin temperature. If the skin is cold, shivering begins at a relatively high central temperature. Conversely, if the skin is warmed, the onset of shivering is delayed until the central temperature drops considerably lower. The most effective way of preventing postoperative shivering is to keep the skin warm!

Tip:

Use of a forced air warming blanket can dramatically decrease the incidence and severity of shivering.

Alpha-2 adrenergic agonists such as clonidine appear to have a specific anti-shivering effect. Given as a premedication, clonidine can substantially prevent shivering after operation.

Pethidine (meperidine in the US) is the only opioid with substantial anti-shivering activity. But to be effective, you have to give a relatively large dose — 25 to 50 mg. Watch out for respiratory depression!

R N Sladen, New York, USA

Hypothermia

In the severely hypothermic patient (e.g. near drowning in a frozen pond), surface warming may not only be ineffective in rewarming the core, but it may increase cutaneous blood flow at the expense of the vital organs. Core rewarming may be accomplished by warm gastric lavage or peritoneal dialysis.

Caveat:

If you are rewarming a hypothermic patient by putting warm fluids into the stomach do not use oesophagal temperature. It will be falsely high. Similarly, if rewarming using peritoneal dialysis do not try and measure core temperature in the rectum.

G R Park, Cambridge, UK

CHAPTER 11

METABOLIC PROBLEMS

Unexplained acidosis

The differential diagnosis of metabolic acidosis may present a challenge.

Tip:

The first step is to calculate the anion gap: $([Na] + [K]) - ([Cl] + [HCO_3^-])$.

If the anion gap is <12 mEq/L, the most likely cause in an ICU patient is hyperchloremic (excess chloride administration), diarrhea or renal tubular acidosis (excess bicarbonate loss).

If the anion gap is ≥ 15 mEq/L, the cause may be lactic acid, ketoacids or non-volatile acids (phosphates and sulphates, which accumulate in acute renal failure).

If none of these fit the bill think of poisoning (methanol, ethylene glycol, salicylates).

K E Gunning, Cambridge, UK
R N Sladen, New York, USA

Potassium and pH

There is a very close relationship between serum potassium and pH. Extracellular acidosis (an increase in extracellular hydrogen ion) results in intracellular movement of hydrogen along the concentration gradient, in exchange for potassium. Alkalosis has the reverse effect.

Tip:

An acute change in pH of 0.1 is associated with an acute change in serum potassium of 0.5 mEq/L.

This has a number of clinical ramifications.

For example, in a mechanically ventilated patient with hyperkalemia (e.g. serum potassium 6.0 mEq/L), hyperventilation to increase the pH from 7.35 to 7.50 could decrease serum potassium by ($1.5 \times 0.5 =$ 0.75 mEq/L), i.e. from 6.0 to 5.25 mEq/L.

A patient has a metabolic acidosis with a pH of 7.20. The serum potassium is 4.0 mEq/L.

Question: What is the patient's true potassium status?

Answer: Hypokalemic.
If the pH were corrected to 7.40 the serum potassium would be 3.0 mEq/L.

R N Sladen, New York, USA

CHAPTER 12

RADIOLOGY

"Step one"

Tip:

Always stand at least a metre away from the film. You will get a much better overview. It does not prevent you from focusing on one area afterwards.

M L Pepperman, Leicester, UK

Reviewing the chest X-ray

It may be difficult to identify fractured ribs on a chest X-ray.

Tip:

If you are looking for broken ribs, turn the X-ray upside down (apex pointing down): the optical illusion makes the ribs stand out and fractures easier to see!

P Lawler, Middlesbrough, UK

Pneumothorax is one of the most important complications that must be detected by chest X-ray review, especially in patients on positive pressure ventilation, who are at risk of tension pneumothorax. A pneumothorax may not be seen on a supine chest X-ray. This is because the lungs are stiff and do not collapse.

Tip:

In a pneumothorax, the edge of the lung is usually marked by a fine white line beyond which there is a darker field without lung markings. If there is no fine white line what you are seeing is more likely to be a skin fold or bone edge.

Look for the "deep sulcus sign" — a dark shadow without lung markings that projects below the costophrenic angle.

Ask for a repeat chest X-ray: stress that it should be upright, and deeply penetrated. It'll help. A lung edge as seen in a classical pneumothorax is usually only apparent if the pneumothorax is large. In a smaller pneumothorax the air lies anteriorly. This results in a classic radiological appearance with a black line outlining the cardiac border on the left or right. This appearance is the result of air in this "gutter".

A lateral decubitus chest X-ray may show an anterior pneumothorax.

R N Sladen, New York, USA
G R Park, Cambridge, UK
K E Gunning, Cambridge, UK

It may be difficult to sort out whether the uniform opacity of one lung field is a pleural effusion, collapse or consolidation.

Tip:

Do another X-ray with the patient in the lateral position, with the suspect side up and shoot through. If the haziness is effusion, it will not disappear into the hilar shadow. Other problems may be disclosed.

P Lawler, Middlesbrough, UK

Caveat:

There is no such thing as "upper lobe diversion" in a supine film. Upper lobe diversion in an upright film indicates that the left atrial pressure is sufficient to back up the venous flow to a blood column height of about 20 cm — from the hilum to the apex — the diagnosis of heart failure in ICU is not that!

P Lawler, Middlesbrough, UK

Pericardial effusion may be difficult to rule out on a chest X-ray

Tip:

Most patients in ICU have a pulse rate of about 100 beats/min. X-ray exposures may be long enough to allow the heart border to move significantly. If the heart borders are sharply demarcated, consider a pericardial effusion.

P Lawler, Middlesbrough, UK

Increased intrathoracic pressure predisposes to pulmonary barotrauma

Tip:

The diagnosis of raised intrathoracic pressure can sometimes be made on the chest X-ray. In such patients the cuff of the endotracheal tube will commonly be visible as a dark shadow. This occurs in patients with increased intrathoracic pressure because the pressure in the cuff needed to produce an airtight seal is also increased and therefore the volume of air in the cuff is increased to a level where the cuff is visible.

M P Shelly, Manchester, UK

Air under the diaphragm

Air under the diaphragm is pathognomic of a perforated abdominal viscus, which may be clinically silent.

Caveat:

Subdiaphragmatic air is expected after laparotomy.

In severe pulmonary barotrauma, air may extend from the mediastinum (pneumomediastinum) into the abdominal cavity and mimic the sign of perforation. In severe cases an entire pneumoperitoneum may develop, outlining all viscera on X-ray.

G R Park, Cambridge, UK
R N Sladen, New York, USA

CHAPTER 13

RENAL SYSTEM

Anuria

Acute renal failure is usually associated with oliguria, not anuria.

Tip:

If a patient becomes anuric, check that the catheter is not blocked, or in the wrong orifice!

K E Gunning, Cambridge, UK

Urinalysis

This is an invaluable, non-invasive cheap test that should be done every day in critically ill patients.

Tip:

Some of the information it can give includes:

Specific gravity:	are the tubules working? is the patient hypovolaemic?
pH:	an acid urine in the presence of a metabolic alkalosis may be a good indicator of total body potassium depletion
Blood:	renal trauma
	immune diseases (Goodpasture's syndrome, vasculitis)
Protein:	nephritis
Glucose:	excessive glucose administration inadequate insulin administration faulty blood glucose measurement resulting in hyperglycaemia being missed.
Bilirubin:	haemolysis

G R Park, Cambridge, UK

Oliguria

It is important to detect oliguria early so that appropriate treatment can be given before there is sustained injury to the kidney.

Tip:

Do not be content with urine volumes of 0.5 mL/kg/h in sick patients, aim for 1 mL/kg/h.

Set limits for two hours of urine production (unless clinically inappropriate). If hypovolaemia has developed over two hours the response to rapid volume replacement is clear and fluid management easily modified.

K E Gunning, Cambridge, UK
M J Lindop, Cambridge, UK

Bedside creatinine clearance

The most sensitive measure of changing renal function is not the serum creatinine, but the creatinine clearance. After all, if one cross-clamped the renal artery and measured the serum creatinine, it would be normal, in the face of a zero glomerular filtration rate (GFR). It would take several days before the serum creatinine reached a new steady state that represented a zero GFR. Serum creatinine represents the equilibrium between creatinine production and excretion.

Creatinine clearance is calculated by UV/P, where U is the urine creatinine in mg/dL, V is the urine flow rate in mL/min and P is the serum creatinine in mg/dL.

The term "UV", i.e. urine creatinine times urine flow rate, represents the creatinine excretion rate. It is THIS that changes rapidly with changing GFR.

Caveat:

Serum creatinine underestimates the degree of renal insufficiency in the following situations:

- Anyone with renal insufficiency but a GFR >50 mL/min, because serum creatinine doesn't start to rise until GFR falls below 50 mL/min.
- Cachexia — because creatinine production is so low. Serum creatinine may rise only when GFR falls below 25 mL/min in some patients.
- After surgery in patients who have received a lot of fluid. A 10–15% increase in total body water results in dilution of serum creatinine by an equivalent amount.

Tip:

The most useful means of estimating GFR at the bedside is a two hour creatinine clearance. There is nothing about clearance that mandates a 24 hr urine collection, particularly when there is a Foley catheter in place, which largely eliminates error due to urine retention. As long as the collection is carefully timed and urine flow is >30 mL/hr, a collection as short as 2 hr will give reasonable data.

R N Sladen, New York, USA

Rhabdomyolysis

Of all the causes of acute renal failure in the ICU rhabdomyolysis is probably the most preventable, because the patient at risk can be identified early and renal protection is easy and reliable.

Tip:

Rhabdomyolysis does not only occur after crush injury. Factors predisposing to rhabdomyolysis include prolonged immobilization (e.g. undetected drug overdose), fever, myoclonus and seizures, and compartment syndrome. Renal injury is always far more likely to occur if the patient is dehydrated and hypovolemic.

Compartment syndrome occurs any time there is a combination of ischemia + tissue edema in an enclosed space. For example, after coronary artery bypass grafting (CABG) surgery, a not uncommon situation is placement of an intraaortic balloon pump in an atherosclerotic femoral artery (ischemia) on the leg from which the vein was stripped (tissue edema).

Myoglobinemic renal injury is much more likely to occur in a young, heavily muscled healthy young person than an old, cachectic patient with renal insufficiency. The former has lots of muscle to release myoglobin and a normal GFR to deliver it to the tubules.

Although a positive urine myoglobin is the earliest warning sign, it may be negative in early rhabdomyolysis because myoglobin is so rapidly cleared by the kidney.

Measurement of creatinine phosphokinase (CPK) is a useful means of estimating the degree of rhabdomyolysis. I have seldom seen renal injury occur when the CPK is less than 10,000 IU/L. Serial CPK levels (q8–12 hr) can tell you whether rhabdomyolysis is still getting worse, or is resolving.

There is good animal evidence that keeping the urine pH >6.0 protects the kidneys from the nephrotoxic effect of myoglobin by preventing its conversion to acid ferrihematin. This can easily be accomplished by adding one or two ampoules of sodium bicarbonate per liter to the maintenance fluid.

The key to renal protection is an expanded intravascular volume and high tubular flow. Provide a maintenance iv flow of 150–250 mL/hr. If that doesn't cause a diuresis (urine flow ≥100 mL/hr) add mannitol 6.25 g every six hours. If that doesn't do it, add furosemide 10–20 mg iv after the mannitol.

R N Sladen, New York, USA

Raised intra-abdominal pressure and oliguria

When the intra-abdominal pressure is markedly elevated by active bleeding, the renal vein pressure rises and progressive oliguria and renal failure results unless the abdomen is decompressed.

Tip:

An easy way to indirectly measure the intra-abdominal pressure is as follows:

1. Inject 50–100 mL sterile saline into the bladder through an indwelling Foley catheter.
2. Clamp the tubing of the drainage bag with a standard surgical clamp.
3. Connect the tubing to the Foley catheter.
4. Release the clamp to fill the tubing, then reapply the clamp.
5. Insert a size 16 French needle through the culture port of the tubing, proximal to the clamp.
6. Connect the needle via small-gauge tubing to a manometer or transducer.
7. Zero the transducer to the top of symphysis pubis, and read the pressure.

If the intra-abdominal pressure is greater than 20 mmHg, surgical decompression of the abdominal distension may be needed to relieve the oliguria and reverse the renal failure.

R N Sladen, New York, USA

Diuresis in patients with low GFR

Patients with oliguria who have a low GFR are "resistant" to loop diuretics such as furosemide (Lasix) because of impaired delivery to the tubules. This is not due to decreased filtration of the diuretic by the glomerulus, but decreased active transport into the tubular lumen at the proximal tubule.

Tip:

Try a "triple-decker intravenous sandwich":

- 500 mg of hydrochlorthiazide
- followed in 10 min by 12.5 g of human albumin
- followed in another 10 min by 200 mg of furosemide

Loop diuretics act at the thick ascending loop of Henle. Further downstream, the distal tubule can compensate by increasing sodium reabsorption. The thiazide diuretic hydrochlorthiazide inhibits this. Administration of albumin increases delivery of the loop diuretic to the tubules.

This is the most potent combination I have found.

D MacGregor, Winston-Salem, North Carolina, USA

CHAPTER 14

GENERAL

Notes

Tip:

When making an entry in the notes write the day of the week as well as the date and time. When thinking back, most people think in days of the week rather than the date. Not only is this useful at the bedside it can be invaluable when dealing with a complaint or in court.

G R Park, Cambridge, UK

Multiple teams

Tip:

When a patient is under the care of multiple clinical and support teams there's always someone who disagrees fundamentally with current management. Every so often it will be you. Never criticize or spell out the incompetence of others in the notes or to relatives. Always write down the evidence in favour of your view. Always document your offer to discuss the matter with the other party. It's never worth getting angry — it is the patient who will suffer.

M Farrington, Cambridge, UK

Nursing staff

Tip:

Nursing staff have much important information to impart to the doctor only some of which will need acting upon. It is important that the nursing staff are aware that the information has registered with the doctor and I find that a "NOTED: NO ACTION" response helps clarify this point and stops the same information being repeatedly given. A similar response of "MASTERLY INACTIVITY" can also convey that taking no action is a considered treatment option and not one of omission.

A White, Milton Keynes, UK

Death

Tip:

A good death is a fitting end to a good life. Doctors caring for the critically ill should never forget the need for compassion, humanity and the realization that at some time death is inevitable. Technology should not be used to prolong dying.

G R Park, Cambridge, UK

Importance of infection

Tip:

Any patient referred to the ICU from a surgical ward with a provisional diagnosis of pneumonia, pulmonary embolism or myocardial infarction has abdominal sepsis until proven otherwise.

G Skowronski, Australia

Thoughts

Tip:

If it can't be done the way it should be done, it should be done the way it can be done.

J L van der Spoel, Netherlands
D F Zandstra, Netherlands

Transferring patients

Tip:

If the patient is receiving an infusion of a diuretic that can be stopped and is ready to be transferred to another area leave the infusion going, let the other area stop the infusion. Then if the urine output goes down the reason will be obvious. Alternatively, stop the infusion and keep the patient a little longer, treat the oliguria and then discharge the patient.

G R Park, Cambridge, UK

Aspiration of ascitic fluid — use of a Z-track approach

Tip:

In patients with massive ascites, use a Z-track technique for paracentesis so that you limit the chance of a continuing leak.

G R Park, Cambridge, UK

Education and research

Tip:

To get teaching points or inclusion criteria for a research project widely disseminated put a brief summary on a sticky label. Most computers will be able to print a sheet of these. They can then be stuck on the telephone base. People tend to read these when not talking on the telephone. In addition, the whole protocol can be printed on a large poster. This can then be stuck on the back of the toilet door. You will have most people's undivided attention at some time or another. However, print off several — graffiti artists are found in all walks of life, even in the ICU!

G R Park, Cambridge, UK

Breaking bad news (1)

Tip:

Occasionally, this has to be done immediately because of a rapid deterioration in the patient's condition. More usually, it can be done as a planned interview. When it can be, it is best done as a pre-arranged formal appointment. This allows the relatives to arrive concentrating solely on the interview. If suddenly "sprung" on the relatives, then their minds are likely to be thinking about other things such as whether the time on the parking meter will expire, or whether the children will be collected from school on time. It also allows the relatives time to get their thoughts together and ask any questions they want to.

G R Park, Cambridge, UK

Breaking bad news (2)

Tip:

Before interviewing patients or their relatives prepare yourself and your environment. You should know who you are seeing, any background to the interview and what you hope to achieve from it. The environment should be arranged so that you are able to see all the people in the room. Sources of interruptions such as telephones should be disconnected and any useful extras, such as boxes of tissues, should be in place.

M P Shelly, Manchester, UK

CHAPTER 15

NUTRITION

Nasogastric tubes that keep being "removed"

Most patients do not remove tubes placed with the "bridle" technique. This should not be used as a routine. The patient requires sedation for insertion of the tube.

Tip:

- First sedate the patient
- Thread about 30 cm of green bubble tubing into one nasal passage and a smaller tube or thread through the other
- Tie one to the other, and pull the green tubing back through the other nostril: the green tubing has now lassoed the nasal septum
- The nasogastric tube must now be inserted through whichever nostril is easiest
- When satisfactorily positioned in the stomach, the tube can be super-glued to the nasogastric tube, most easily by cutting a slot in each green tube: this can be sleeved around the nasogastric tube with or without overlap

P Lawler, Middlesbrough, UK

The gut won't work

Tip:

Try:

1. Erythromycin 250 mg iv 6 hrly
2. Metoclopramide 10 mg iv 8 hrly
3. Cisapride* 10 mg 8 hrly NGT — but this cannot be combined with fluconazole or erythromycin (prolonged QT)

P Lawler, Middlesbrough, UK

*Cisapride has been withdrawn in the UK and USA because of the risk of potentially fatal arrythmias.

No bowels sound does not mean the gut is not working

Tip:

Bowel sounds are not a reliable indicator of gastrointestinal function in critical illness. Bowel sounds require the presence of movement, intestinal contents and intralumenal air. Normally air is swallowed and ventilated patients, particularly if receiving neuromuscular blocking agents, do not swallow air. Because of this bowel sounds may be absent in patients whose gastrointestinal tract is not working normally.

M P Shelly, Manchester, UK